Dr. Douglas Markham is the author of *Total Health* and *Beyond Atkins* (coming soon from Pocket Books), and the founder of www.total-healthdoc.com, an online weight-loss and wellness management system that has helped thousands of people lose weight and achieve a healthy lifestyle. He has appeared on CNN's *Larry King Live,* where he announced the launch of his HEALTH Across America Tour, a national obesity-prevention public education campaign that targeted America's twenty-five "fattest cities." He lives in Southern California.

PRAISE FOR DR. DOUG

"[He] is America's answer to our obesity and health crisis."
—Larry King, host of CNN's *Larry King Live*

"Dr. Doug has created the perfect healthy balance between Atkins and [the] Zone diet. His system helped me lose weight and increase my energy levels dramatically!"
—Jack Canfield, coauthor, *Chicken Soup for the Soul* series

"My family and I follow [Dr. Doug's] well-balanced principles."
—John Schneider, actor/director, and star
of the WB television series *Smallville*

"Dr. Doug's *Total Health* program can literally help save people's lives!"
—Dr. Henry Heimlich, physician/humanitarian, developer of the Heimlich Maneuver and founder of the Heimlich Institute

Don't miss Dr. Doug's groundbreaking guide to healthy low-carb eating
BEYOND ATKINS
Coming soon from Pocket Books

Books by Dr. Douglas J. Markham

Low-Carb Cocktails

*Beyond Atkins: A Healthier, More Balanced Approach
to a Low-Carbohydrate Way of Eating*

Available from Pocket Books

Low-Carb Cocktails

Delicious Alcoholic and Nonalcoholic Beverages
for All Low-Carbohydrate Lifestyles

Dr. Douglas J. Markham

POCKET BOOKS

New York London Toronto Sydney

POCKET BOOKS, a division of Simon & Schuster, Inc.
1230 Avenue of the Americas, New York, NY 10020

ISBN: 1-4165-0387-0

First Pocket Books trade paperback edition November 2004

10 9 8 7 6 5 4 3 2 1

POCKET and colophon are registered trademarks
of Simon & Schuster, Inc.

Manufactured in the United States of America

For information regarding special discounts for bulk purchases,
please contact Simon & Schuster Special Sales at
1-800-456-6798 or business@simonandschuster.com.

I dedicate this book to the human race.

*I pray that the contents of this book contribute
to the joy, happiness and enhanced quality of life of families,
loved-ones, friends and co-workers throughout the world
who gather together to celebrate their lives in
peace, harmony and prosperity.*

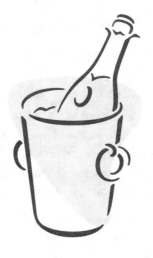

Acknowledgments

The completion of this book would not have been possible without the support of the following people:

Thanks to my wife, 'Drea, for her continued love and support for my numerous projects.

Many thanks to Dr. John Skhal, PharmD, for his support, suggestions and sampling help as a true connoisseur of fine wines and low-carb cocktails.

Tons of thanks to Louise Burke, President/Publisher of Pocket Books; Liate Stehlik, Vice President/Associate Publisher; and Christina Boys, Associate Editor, for their vision and support of this fun and exciting project.

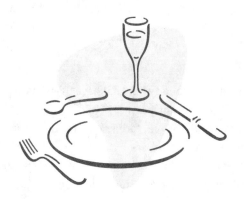

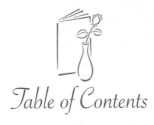

Table of Contents

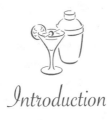

Introduction

*A*fter consulting with thousands of patients for weight loss and wellness in my private practice and online at www.total-healthdoc.com, I saw the need to offer individuals more low-carb options. Even though I've always recommended healthier protein and carbohydrate choices through my Total Health program, I'm not a purest. I'm a realist! Not every person, including myself, is going to shop in health food stores one hundred percent of the time.

That's why people need alternate food options, from fast-food and low-carb desserts to alcoholic beverages. I've always told my patients and online weight loss members to be realistic when embarking on their weight loss and wellness programs. Life goes on during their journeys to their target weights and long after they've reached them. Whether it's a birthday, a retirement party, a wedding or an after-work get-together, there's always something. People need options.

There's an estimated 59 million Americans presently following low-carbohydrate principles, and they all want more options. As a result, the skyrocketing demand for low-carb foods and snacks has created many more great-tasting options. Congratulations fellow

low-carb followers, your time has come and it's here to stay! Hence, I present you with *Low-Carb Cocktails*.

Because I enjoy an occasional alcoholic beverage myself, I've been perfecting low-carb cocktail options for some time now. Of course, like most things in life, we must exercise a certain amount of moderation, especially regarding alcohol consumption. That's why we'll be discussing some of the effects of alcohol and how our body metabolizes it.

It's my sincere wish for you to enjoy the wonderfully delicious low-carb cocktails you're about to experience in this book. Whether you're on your way to your weight loss goals or just want to maintain without all the sugar, this book is for you.

Oh, by the way! More exciting news! This book also includes many mouth-watering protein-rich snacks sure to be the hit of any low-carb cocktail party!

So get out the blender, call your friends, and celebrate! Remember, you deserve to be both healthy and happy.

One Final Note: The low-carb cocktail program is subject to modifications based on the developments of new recipes, suggested alcohol choices, sugar-free sweeteners, syrups, mixers and low-carb products. This book contains information that is current at the time of printing. For the latest updates and information on new products, existing products and links on where to buy these products online or at various retail outlets, visit our website at: www.lowcarbcocktails.com.

Be safe, have fun and drink responsibly!

Yours in Total Health,
Dr. Doug

Principles of the Low-Carb Lifestyle

$\mathcal{T}$o fully understand the principles of a low-carb lifestyle we must look at the main reason we crave food, which has to do with our brain's physiological need for sugar, or what is called the *dietary hormonal connection*. There are two dietary hormones called insulin and glucagon that are secreted from the pancreas. Insulin, which our bodies produce when we eat carbohydrates, causes our body to store fat. Glucagon, which is produced when we eat protein, causes our body to burn fat. The key to why low-carb dieting works is *blood sugar regulation*. In other words, the kind of food you eat, how much you eat and when you eat determine whether or not your body is going to store or burn fat. Therefore the object is to produce less fat-storing insulin by lowering our carb consumption, and more fat-burning glucagon by eating more protein.

Let's take a look at an ordinary breakfast that many of us have probably eaten over the past fifteen to twenty years. If you're not already a low-carb follower, you might start out with an 8:00 A.M. bowl of oatmeal. Although oats are virtually void of fat, they're still a form of carbohydrate that converts into sugar fairly rapidly.

Now let's say you add a sliced banana on top of your oatmeal. The banana is a good source of potassium, but it's high in natural fruit sugar that also converts into sugar very rapidly. You may also accompany your bowl of oatmeal with a glass of fruit juice. And what is fruit juice? It's almost 100 percent fruit sugar in liquid form!

So other than the splash of milk you added to your oatmeal, you ate a 100 percent carbohydrate breakfast. And what do carbohydrates do? They convert into sugar. At first this makes your brain very happy. The brain is a sugar hog, due to its need for glucose, which gives it energy. Therefore it consumes about two-thirds of the circulating carbohydrates (sugar) in the blood.

But when blood sugars are elevated, insulin is released from the pancreas. Insulin is responsible for taking our blood sugars through our cell walls for energy. About sixty to ninety grams of sugars are stored in the liver, and about two hundred to three hundred grams are stored in our muscles. So once our cells have used the blood sugars for energy and these storage areas are full, the extra blood sugars are stored via insulin in our adipose tissue, or fat.

This is the same way we fatten the pigs and cows in my home state of Wisconsin with carbohydrates such as grain. Unfortunately some of us are more predisposed to weight gain than others, and this is how excessive carbohydrate consumption translates into excessive weight gain.

Now what happens once your body burns all the glucose and your blood sugar starts to drop around 10:00 A.M.? You start to nod off, get hungry and reach for your stash of candy in your bottom desk drawer. This rapidly satisfies your brain's need for sugar, your energy levels shoot back up and you've successfully taken a ride on what is called the *blood sugar roller coaster*—going from low levels of blood sugar and low energy to high levels of blood sugar and high energy, never achieving those sustained energy levels that we're all looking for.

Now don't get depressed! Fortunately there's the counterbalancing hormone I mentioned earlier called glucagon. When the level of glucagon is high enough in the blood, it will stimulate the liver to release some of its stored sugars into the blood. This satisfies our brain's cravings for sugar.

Dietary protein stimulates the release of glucagon from the pancreas. So instead of eating the high-carbohydrate oatmeal breakfast, you may consider choosing an egg white omelet with reduced-fat cheese, in addition to carbohydrates in the form of fiber-rich fruit like apples and oranges, which don't covert into sugar too rapidly. The next time 10:00 A.M. rolls around, the glucagon will have stimulated the release of some of the stored sugars in the liver into the blood. This satisfies your brain's cravings for sugar, so you won't be reaching for your candy stash.

By eating every three and a half to four hours, you will burn stored sugars and fat for energy rather than taking another ride on the blood sugar roller coaster. There's not a pharmaceutical company in the world that will produce a diet pill as effective as the kind of food you eat, how much you eat and when you eat it!

Since 1996 I've consulted with thousands of patients on a more balanced approach to a low-carbohydrate way of eating, to develop the Total Health eating plan. The Total Health Plan is based on a protein-rich, favorable-carbohydrate way of eating.

Now even though excessive carbohydrate consumption is the major culprit in weight gain, we still don't want to disregard portion control and the fat content of our protein choices. This is also where I differ from the Atkins type of high-protein diet plans. They work well in the short term, but they are too unbalanced for overall long-term health.

The Total Health Plan outlines your daily protein requirements based on your body frame size and allows fruit as a carbohydrate choice in the initial stages of weight loss. The details of the Total Health Plan are available in my new book, *Beyond Atkins.*

Just like our food choices, we should be aware of the protein and carbohydrate content of what we drink, and choose low-carb options whenever possible. You can follow a low-carb lifestyle, and still have fun!

How to Party Without Adding Pounds

Much of this book is geared toward hosting a low-carb cocktail party, in addition to letting you know what you need to have on hand for preparing low-carb cocktails at home. But what happens when you find yourself attending someone else's party, or you meet for drinks with friends at a local bar, restaurant or cocktail lounge after work?

Consider the following helpful tips:

- Choose drinks with a sugar-free mixer like rum and diet cola, whisky or tequila with diet 7 UP, a vodka or gin gimlet on the rocks or strained in a cocktail glass, a martini, a Scotch and water or Scotch on the rocks, a fine sipping tequila.
- If you're attending someone's party, take your own bottle of diet tonic for a gin or vodka tonic, take packets of Crystal Light® lemonade for sweet 'n' sour or margarita mix. This also works in a cocktail lounge setting. You can put the Crystal Light® lemonade packets in your pocket or purse and add some to a glass of water.

Order a shot of tequila and a glass of ice, and mix your own sugar-free margarita on the rocks!

- When attending a party, avoid snacks like chips. Choose a handful of nuts instead, which are a great source of mixed protein and carbs. Go for the cheese and vegetable platter. Have some cheese with radishes or celery with cream cheese. If there's assorted deli meats, consider wrapping a piece of cheese with some deli ham and dip it in mustard.

- If you're at happy hour with friends or coworkers after work and it's time to eat, order protein appetizers like shrimp with cocktail sauce, buffalo wings or a seared ahi appetizer.

See how simple it really is when you use a little creative thinking and planning ahead?

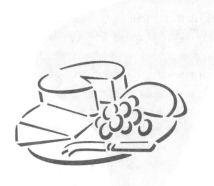

Understanding the Types
of Alcohol

*A*lcoholic beverages are now consumed by approximately 70 percent of all American adults and by 80 percent of all college students. Per capita, Americans consume about 8.7 liters of ethanol per year. Canadians consume about 10.8 liters per person, with 73 percent of Canadians over eighteen drinking occasionally. In other English-speaking countries, over 90 percent of university-aged students drink.

Only about 30 percent of North Americans choose not to drink, often because they don't like the taste, they choose not to for religious reasons or illness, or they're recovering alcoholics. Otherwise, most Americans enjoy the occasional use of alcohol as a socially acceptable and enjoyable adult beverage option.

Alcohol (ethanol) in alcoholic beverages generally comes in three forms: wines, beers and distilled beverages. Wines are made from fermenting the juices of a variety of fruits, honey and some grains. Beers are made by cooking and fermenting complex sugars or grains such as corn, rice, barley, etc., which are then flavored with hops, giving beer its bitter taste.

Distilled spirits such as vodka, whisky, gin, rum and tequila are made from distilling the alcohol from wines. Sherry and port are wines fortified with brandy or other distilled spirits in order to increase alcohol content or to stop the fermentation process. Liqueurs or cordials are made with sweetened spirits distilled from fruits, seeds, herbs and peels. The process of fermentation and distillation produces small amounts of chemical substances called congeners. They cause the characteristic taste and smell of a particular distilled spirit.

Most beers contain from 2 to 6 percent alcohol by volume. Wines contain 12 to 21 percent alcohol by volume, and distilled spirits contain 40 to 50 percent alcohol by volume. Proof is the alcoholic content of a spirit determined in the United States by doubling the percentage of alcohol. An 80-proof liquor, for example, has 40 percent alcohol content. There's approximately the same amount of alcohol in a twelve-ounce bottle of beer, five-ounce glass of wine, and a shot of whisky, all of which are equivalent to about three-quarters of an ounce of ethanol.

Alcohol is sometimes considered a food, with each gram of alcohol containing seven calories. These are often called empty calories because they have no nutritional value. A half ounce of alcohol contains approximately 100 calories, but the sugars found in most drinks, such as beer and wine, give higher calories to each average-sized drink. Eight ounces of wine contain approximately 270 calories, a twelve-ounce bottle of beer contains about 170 calories, and two ounces of whiskey contain about 140 calories.

As low-carb followers, most of our discussions related to the physical effects of alcohol will be related to its carbohydrate content and how it affects our blood sugars. Distilled alcohol (ethanol) doesn't directly raise blood sugar (glucose) levels. That's why we recommend hard liquor or distilled alcohols either straight or with sugar-free mixers over beers and wines. Beers and wines contain natural sugars or carbohydrates that convert into sugar and can eventually end up around the midsection of our bodies in the form of stored fat!

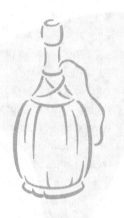

The Physical Effects of Alcohol

*T*he effect of alcohol on blood sugar levels depends on both the amount and types of alcohol ingested and its relationship to food intake. The same precautions that apply to alcohol consumption for the general public apply to persons with diabetes. However, in diabetics who are taking insulin, alcohol may cause low blood sugars (hypoglycemia).

The liver is the organ that metabolizes (breaks down) alcohol, however, it does so slowly. A man weighing 150 pounds will require about two hours to metabolize one ounce of alcohol. Our livers store about sixty to ninety grams of stored sugars. During times of low blood sugar, these stored sugars can be released for use. However, when the liver is breaking down alcohol, it's too busy to release the stored sugar, and blood sugars may drop too low.

For most individuals, blood glucose levels are not affected by moderate use of alcohol. For people using insulin to control diabetes, up to two alcoholic beverages (one twelve-ounce beer, five-ounce glass of wine, or one and a half ounces of distilled spirits) can be consumed with their regular daily meal plans. Food should not be omitted because of the possibility of alcohol-induced hypoglycemia.

Caution: Responsible drinking may mean not drinking at all, particularly when a person is suffering from illness, taking medications, is pregnant, or diabetic with blood glucose levels that are out of control. Always consult with a physician before consuming alcoholic beverages.

Choosing the Right Wines

Due to the higher carbohydrate content of most beers and wine, we will be recommending most of our low-carb drink options in the form of distilled spirits either straight, on-the-rocks (over ice) or with sugar-free mixers.

Unfortunately there are few low-carb wines on the market, but the good news for wine lovers is that most unsweetened wines are naturally low in carbs. Some wineries are even beginning to add labels listing calorie and carbohydrate counts. White wines contain approximately one gram of carbs per four ounces, and red wines contain two grams per four-ounce serving.

This is even better news for white-wine lovers because you can have twice as much for the same amount of carbs. Although don't interpret this as a license to drink too much wine. Remember to exercise moderation in all things!

Choosing the Right Beer

When it comes to choosing the appropriate beer, there's a more significant difference between certain brands. Most standard domestic beers contain about 12.5 grams of carbs per twelve-ounce serving. Therefore most beer lovers are going to have a harder time following the low-carb lifestyle.

Several beer manufacturers are now advertising low-carb beers, but you'll find that many of the light beers presently on the market contain about the same amount of carbs and calories as the new low-carb or ultra-light beers. Therefore the beer connoisseur can usually stay with their favorite-tasting choice of light beer.

The following list contains some of the most popular brands of light and ultra-light beers for a comparison of carbs and calories based on a twelve-ounce serving:

Beer	Carbohydrates	Calories
Amstel Light	5 grams	95
Aspen Edge	2.6 grams	94
Bud Light	6.6 grams	110
Coors Light	5 grams	102
Corona Light	5 grams	105
Labatt's Blue Light	8 grams	111
Michelob Ultra	2.6 grams	95
Miller Lite	3.2 grams	96
Milwaukee's Best Light	3.5 grams	98
Natural Light	3.2 grams	95
Rock Green Light	2.6 grams	92
Samuel Adams Light	9.7 grams	124

The Responsible Use of Alcohol

We're a society of social drinkers. Responsible drinking in social situations, from celebrations to cocktail parties, should have some guidelines to help you get the most from your low-carb cocktail experience. As mentioned earlier, responsible drinking may mean not drinking at all. Whether you're on medications or the designated driver, *you never have to feel sorry about having an excuse not to drink.*

The following tips are designed to help you drink responsibly and derive enhanced enjoyment from your low-carb cocktail experience:

1. **Know your limit.** If you don't know your limit, test it out at home in the presence of a responsible adult. Most people will find that no more than about a drink and a half per hour will keep them in control and avoid intoxication.

2. **Don't drink on an empty stomach.** Before drinking in a social situation, it's a good idea to eat or snack on protein-rich foods such as nuts and cheese, which slow the absorption of alcohol.

3. **Savor your drink.** Don't gulp your drink. Enjoy the pleasure of the tastes and smells of various flavors.
4. **Cultivate fine taste.** Make quality alcohol choices. Getting the most out of your low-carb cocktail experience means choosing high-quality liquor choices. That's why it's important to choose premium brands as your preferred choices in the Low-Carb Cocktail Recipes section.
5. **Choose a designated driver.** The safest rule for drinking and driving is to *not drink and drive!* Use designated drivers who don't drink at the party, or call a taxi, and make sure everyone gets home safely.

Note: Below are general guidelines of how long it takes people of different body sizes to metabolize alcoholic beverages. This chart should not be used as a guide to test your drinking limit! If you drink, DON'T DRIVE!

HOW MANY HOURS IT TAKES TO METABOLIZE ALCOHOL

Body Weight (in pounds)	Number of Drinks					
	1	2	3	4	5	6
100–119	0	3	6	10	13	16
120–139	0	2	5	8	10	12
140–159	0	2	4	6	8	10
160–179	0	1	3	5	7	9
180–199	0	0	2	4	6	7
200–219	0	0	2	3	4	6
Over 220	0	0	1	3	4	6

THE RESPONSIBLE USE OF ALCOHOL

Responsible Hosting and Bartending Tips

1. **Don't make your drinks too strong.** Make sure the bartender isn't overly generous with the alcohol content of the drinks. Double shots can lead to double trouble! Don't get your guests drunk. Moderation is the key to an enjoyable party atmosphere.

2. **Always keep an adequate supply of nonalcoholic drinks.** It's always a good idea to have nonalcoholic drink options available for guests who don't consume alcohol, have had too much to drink or just want to pace themselves. Refer to the Nonalcoholic Drinks section of this book for a variety of delicious "virgin" cocktails.

3. **Promote snacks.** Push protein-rich snacks such as cheese and nuts, which slow the absorption of alcohol. Always make sure people are eating along with drinking. Refer to the Protein-Rich Low-Carb Snacks section for recipes.

4. **Make a mental note of the number of drinks your guests have consumed.** Keeping tabs on your guests' alcohol consumption is a good idea. It's never considered rude to cut off a guest who's had too much to drink—especially when you're considering their potential health and safety.

5. **Plan activities for your guests.** If your guests have plenty to do, they're less likely to get drunk. Good conversation, food, games, etc., create added fun and healthy diversions for the ultimate low-carb cocktail party.

6. **Bringing your party or social gathering to a close.** It's a good idea to stop serving alcohol and start serving coffee and protein-rich snacks prior to the close of your party. This allows time for your guests to metabolize their prior consumption of alcohol and have a safe trip home.

Stocking Your Low-Carb Cocktail Bar

The following list includes everything you'll need for stocking your low-carb cocktail bar to help to ensure the ultimate pleasurable experience in taste for you and your future low-carb cocktail guests.

Liquor

Since distilled alcohols have "zero" carbs and aren't converted into sugar by the body, it's the number one alcohol choice for a low-carb cocktail with or without a sugar-free mixer.

Premium dry English gin

Jamaican dark rum

Gold rum

Light rum

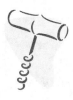

Premium Scotch whisky

Premium Irish whisky

Premium Tennessee whisky

Brandy

Gold tequila

White tequila

Premium vodka

Liqueurs

Due to the high amount of added and natural sugars in liqueurs, we'll be recommending the following sugar-free flavored syrups as the appropriate low-carb alternatives:

Triple sec—*substitute orange sugar-free syrup*

Crème de menthe—*substitute crème de menthe sugar-free syrup*

Kahlúa—*substitute coffee-flavored or* Kahlua® *sugar-free syrup*

Amaretto—*substitute amaretto sugar-free syrup*

Irish cream—*substitute Irish cream sugar-free syrup*

Note: The complete list of recommended sugar-free flavored syrups, including the above mentioned, is located in Sugar-Free Mixers section.

Beer, Wine and Champagne

As previously mentioned, beers and wines all contain carbohydrates that convert into sugar. Therefore the consumption of beer, wine and champagne will have to be more limited for low-carb followers.

The following beer and wine selections are based on lower carbohydrate contents:

Favorite light beer (12 oz = approximately 2.8 grams of carbs)

White wine (4 oz. = 1 gram of carbs)

Red wine (4 oz. = 2 grams of carbs)

Sparkling wine or preferred brand of champagne
(4 oz. = 3.5 grams of carbs)

Note: When consuming beer or wine during the weight loss or maintenance phases of your low-carb diet program, you'll need to count the carbohydrate content of the product you're consuming.

Sugar-Free Mixers

Note: For information on where to buy sugar-free syrups online or at various retail outlets, as well as the latest recommended brands, visit our website at: www.lowcarbcocktails.com.

Coffee

Half & half

Cream (heavy and light)

Diet cola

Diet lemon-lime soda

Diet ginger ale

Seltzer

Water (distilled or spring)

Club soda

Diet tonic

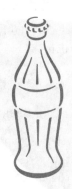

Tabasco sauce

Worcestershire sauce

Bitters

Dry vermouth

Red vermouth

Orgeat *(substitute almond sugar-free syrup)*

Rose's Lime Juice

Orange juice *(substitute Sugar-Free Tang® for orange juice)*

Grapefruit juice *(substitute Crystal Light® Ruby Red Grapefruit for grapefruit juice)*

Cranberry juice (Ocean Spray® Light Cranberry Juice Cocktail)

Pineapple juice *(substitute pineapple sugar-free syrup)*

Grenadine *(substitute cherry sugar-free syrup)*

Simple syrup *(sugar-free)   Note: To make sugar-free simple syrup, mix 4 tablespoons of* Splenda® *sweetener with 4 tablespoons of water in a saucepan. Bring to a slow boil, stirring constantly until sweetener is dissolved. Boil for 1 minute without stirring and allow to cool. Cover and refrigerate until needed.*

Cream of coconut   *Note: To make cream of coconut, mix 3 ounces of coconut sugar-free syrup with 6 ounces of heavy cream in a glass. Stir until well mixed. Cover and refrigerate until needed.*

Sweet 'n' sour mix *(substitute Crystal Light® lemonade for sweet 'n' sour or margarita mix) Note: To make sweet 'n' sour mix, simply double the strength of the recommended amounts of Crystal Light® lemonade for 2 quarts of water to achieve a syrup consistency. Refrigerate until needed.*

Sugar-free syrups come in a wide range of flavors. You may want to add the following flavors to your bar depending on your personal tastes and those of your guests:

Almond sugar-free syrup

Amaretto sugar-free syrup

Banana sugar-free syrup

Blueberry sugar-free syrup

Butter rum sugar-free syrup

Cherry sugar-free syrup

Chocolate sugar-free syrup

Coconut sugar-free syrup

Crème de menthe sugar-free syrup

Eggnog sugar-free syrup

Gingerbread sugar-free syrup

Green apple sugar-free syrup

Hazelnut sugar-free syrup

Irish cream sugar-free syrup

Lemon-lime sugar-free syrup

Lime sugar-free syrup

Orange sugar-free syrup

Peach sugar-free syrup

Peppermint sugar-free syrup

Strawberry sugar-free syrup

Watermelon sugar-free syrup

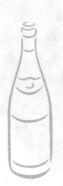

Miscellaneous Ingredients

No low-carb bar would be complete without the following ingredients and garnishes to make your low-carb cocktails come alive! Make sure to include the following:

Olives *(small green pitted olives are the most popular for drinks)*

Cocktail onions *(pearl onions are most commonly used in martinis)*

Cherries *(maraschino cherries make great garnishes for Manhattans or tropical and mixed drinks)*

Lemons *(lemons can be cut into wedges, slices or wheels; the rinds can also be used for twists)*

Limes *(limes can also be cut into wedges, slices, wheels or twists)*

Oranges *(orange slices make a nice decorative and tasty garnish for tropical or exotic drinks)*

Pineapple *(pineapple spears or slices can be added to many tropical drinks, such as piña coladas)*

Nutmeg *(nutmeg can be sprinkled on hot drinks for a tasty garnish)*

Salt *(a coarse salt works best for frosting margarita glasses)*

Sugar (Splenda® *sweetener should be used as an alternative for sugar)*

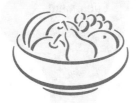

Note: Splenda® is the trade name for sucralose, which is the only calorie-free sweetener made from sugar. It's available in two "tabletop" forms: granular and packet. The granular measures, pours and can be used like real sugar even in cooking and baking. Each packet contains the equivalent of 2 teaspoons of sugar. Sugar substitutes other than Splenda®, such as Equal®, Sweet'n Low®, etc., are also acceptable alternatives to sugar. Personal brand preferences and availability may play a role in what sugar substitute to use when replacing sugar.

Be sure to refer to my new book, *Beyond Atkins,* for a more detailed description of all the artificial sweeteners and sugar substitutes available on the market.

Supplies

Cocktail napkins

Coasters

Straws

Stirrers/Swizzle sticks

Toothpicks *(for garnishes)*

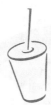

Equipment

Bar spoon *(long handle—a long-handled stainless steel spoon used for mixing and stirring)*

Can/Bottle opener *(a standard can/bottle opener is essential for opening cans and bottles)*

Electric blender *(a powerful electric blender is needed for grinding ice and blending drinks)*

Champagne stopper *(a good champagne stopper will preserve the carbonation of most champagnes for at least twenty-four hours)*

Corkscrew *(the best wine openers are the classic waiter's and wing-type corkscrews)*

Cocktail shaker *(the standard stainless steel shaker has three pieces: a strainer, lid and receptacle)*

Paring knife/Bar knife/Cutting board *(a paring or bar knife and a standard cutting board are handy for cutting and preparing garnishes)*

Ice bucket and Tongs *(the ice bucket is the most appealing way to keep ice at your bar; serve ice with tongs)*

Jigger *(the best jigger is the double-headed stainless steel type that measures 1 and 1½ ounces)*

Measuring cup *(a small 1-cup Pyrex measuring cup is fine for most drink recipes)*

Measuring spoons *(the standard kitchen measuring spoon set is essential)*

Mixing pitcher *(a standard 2-quart pitcher works well for mixing and storing sweet 'n' sour mixes, etc.)*

Saucers *(a coffee cup saucer may be used for salt or sugar substitute to frost the rim of a margarita glass, etc.)*

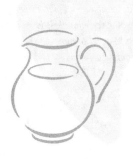

Glassware

The latest and most practical trends have been leaning toward multipurpose glassware. Rather than having a different style of glass for several dozen types of drinks, I suggest the following:

Champagne tulip *(a tall stemmed glass used for champagne or wine; holds 4 to 6 ounces)*

Cocktail glass *(a stemmed glass with sloping sides and a wide mouth that holds from 3 to 6 ounces; they can be used for martinis, Manhattans and many frozen drinks such as margaritas)*

Double old-fashioned glass *(a larger old-fashioned glass that will hold from 14 to 16 ounces—also called a "double rocks" glass; a great multipurpose glass for beer or larger drinks "on the rocks")*

Irish coffee mug *(used for hot drinks and coffee drinks; holds 10 to 12 ounces)*

Old-fashioned glass *(also called a "lowball" or "rocks" glass; ranges in size from 6 to 8 ounces; used for smaller drinks served "on the rocks," and can be used to serve straight shots of liquor if you don't have shot glasses)*

Shot glass *(the standard shot glass comes in many shapes and sizes, ranging from 1 to 2 ounces; the standard shot or jigger is 1½ ounces, and a long shot is 2 ounces)*

Wineglass *(both the red and white wineglasses hold from 6 to 11 ounces; the red wineglass is more rounded than a white wineglass in order to direct the bouquet to the drinker's nose; the wineglass can also be used for frozen or exotic/tropical drinks)*

Low-Carb Cocktails Nutritional Facts

*Y*ou'll notice in the upcoming low-carb drink recipe section that the nutritional facts will only be listing protein, carbohydrates and calories, but because distilled alcohol doesn't contain protein or carbohydrates, most of the drink recipes will have zero protein and zero carbohydrates. The only time you'll note any protein will be with drink recipes that include dairy products. Some of the cocktail mixers will include small amounts of carbohydrates, which will be listed. Garnishes or fruits not blended into drinks won't be counted as carbohydrates in the drink recipes as long as you don't eat them. Some of the mouth-watering fruit flavored martini recipes also contain fruit in the shaker, but the amount of minimal fruit juice strained through won't need to be counted as carbohydrates either.

Distilled alcohols such as vodka, rum, and the like do contain calories. The literal definition of a calorie is the amount of energy or heat it takes to raise the temperature of water one degree Celsius or 1.8 degrees Fahrenheit. The calories on a food package are measured in kilocalories (1,000 calories = 1 kilocalorie). When an exercise chart lists that you burn 100 calories when jogging one mile, it means 100 kilocalories. One gram of carbohydrates equals four calories, one gram of protein equals four calories and one gram of fat equals nine calories. It's going to take more exercise to burn off food or drinks higher in calories. Therefore, excessive caloric intake can lead to weight gain.

Note: The nutritional information in the drink recipes section does not include the garnishes.

Low-Carb Cocktail Recipes

American Blended Whisky Drinks

Algonquin

1¹/₂ ounces blended whisky
¹/₂ ounce dry vermouth
1 ounce pineapple sugar-free syrup

Shake all the ingredients in a shaker with ice and strain into a chilled cocktail glass.

Nutritional Facts: Protein: 0   Carbohydrates: 0   Calories: 106

Aquarius

- 2 ounces blended whisky
- 1 ounce brandy
- 1 ounce cranberry juice (Ocean Spray® Light Cranberry Juice Cocktail)

Shake all the ingredients in a shaker with ice and strain into an old-fashioned glass over crushed ice.

Nutritional Facts: Protein: 0   Carbohydrates: 2.8 grams
Calories: 204

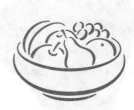

Blue Monday

- 2 ounces Canadian whisky
- 1 ounce blueberry sugar-free syrup
- ½ ounce brandy

Shake all the ingredients in a shaker with ice and strain into a chilled cocktail glass.

Nutritional Facts: Protein: 0   Carbohydrates: 0   Calories: 163.5

Cablegram

2 ounces blended whisky
$\frac{1}{2}$ ounce lemon juice
$\frac{1}{4}$ teaspoon Splenda® sweetener
4 ounces diet ginger ale
Lemon twist

Mix the first three ingredients into a shaker with ice. Strain into a glass filled with crushed ice. Add the diet ginger ale and garnish with the lemon twist.

Nutritional Facts: Protein: 0   Carbohydrates: 1.3 grams
Calories: 132

California Lemonade

2 ounces blended whisky
1 ounce lemon juice
1 teaspoon Splenda® sweetener
4 ounces club soda

Add the first three ingredients to a mixing glass with a scoop of ice. Stir with a long-handled spoon 20 times. Strain into an old-fashioned glass over ice and add the club soda.

Nutritional Facts: Protein: 0   Carbohydrates: 2.6 grams
Calories: 136

Canadian Cocktail

    2 ounces blended whisky
    1 ounce triple sec (substitute orange sugar-free syrup)
    $^1/_2$ teaspoon Splenda® sweetener
    Dash of bitters

Shake all the ingredients in a shaker with ice and strain into a chilled cocktail glass.

Nutritional Facts: Protein: 0   Carbohydrates: 0   Calories: 128

Double Standard Sour

    1 ounce blended whisky
    1 ounce gin
    1 ounce lemon juice
    $^1/_2$ teaspoon Splenda® sweetener
    $^1/_2$ teaspoon grenadine (substitute cherry sugar-free syrup)
    Cherry

Shake all the ingredients in a shaker with ice and strain into a chilled cocktail glass. Garnish with the cherry.

Nutritional Facts: Protein: 0   Carbohydrates: 2.6 grams
Calories: 137

Fancy Whisky

    2 ounces blended whisky
    ½ ounce simple syrup (sugar-free)
    ½ teaspoon triple sec (substitute orange sugar-free syrup)
    Dash of bitters
    Lemon twist

Shake all the ingredients in a shaker with ice and strain into a chilled cocktail glass. Garnish with the lemon twist.

Nutritional Facts: Protein: 0   Carbohydrates: 0   Calories: 128

Houston Hurricane

    1 ounce blended whisky
    1 ounce gin
    1 ounce crème de menthe sugar-free syrup
    3 tablespoons lemon juice

Mix ingredients into a shaker filled with ice. Shake and strain into a chilled cocktail glass.

Nutritional Facts: Protein: 0   Carbohydrates: 3.9 grams
Calories: 141

Imperial Fizz

    2 ounces blended whisky
    1 ounce lemon juice
    $\frac{1}{2}$ teaspoon Splenda® sweetener
    4 ounces club soda

Shake the blended whisky, lemon juice and Splenda® sweetener in a shaker with ice and strain into an old-fashioned glass over crushed ice. Fill the glass with club soda and stir.

Nutritional Facts: Protein: 0   Carbohydrates: 2.6 grams
Calories: 136

Manhattan (dry)

    2 ounces blended whisky
    1 ounce dry vermouth
    Dash of bitters
    Cherry
    Lemon twist

Shake all the ingredients in a shaker with ice and strain into a chilled cocktail glass. Garnish with the cherry and lemon twist.

Nutritional Facts: Protein: 0   Carbohydrates: 0   Calories: 148

Milk Punch

2 ounces blended whisky
2 ounces milk (reduced fat—2%)
1 teaspoon Splenda® sweetener
¼ teaspoon nutmeg

Shake all the ingredients in a shaker with ice and strain into a chilled cocktail glass. Garnish with nutmeg.

Nutritional Facts: Protein: 3 grams   Carbohydrates: 3 grams
Calories: 168

New York Cocktail

2 ounces blended whisky
1 ounce lemon juice
1 teaspoon Splenda® sweetener
½ teaspoon grenadine (substitute sugar-free cherry syrup)
Lemon twist

Shake all the ingredients in a shaker with ice and strain into a chilled cocktail glass. Garnish with the lemon twist.

Nutritional Facts: Protein: 0   Carbohydrates: 2.6 grams
Calories: 136

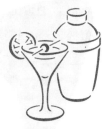

Old-Fashioned

$1/2$ ounce water
1 teaspoon Splenda® sweetener
Several dashes of bitters
3 ounces blended whisky
Cherry

Mix the water, Splenda® sweetener and bitters in an old-fashioned glass. Add whisky and crushed ice and stir. Garnish with the cherry and serve with a swizzle stick.

Nutritional Facts: Protein: 0   Carbohydrates: 0   Calories: 192

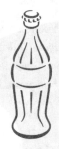

Seven and Seven

$1^1/2$ ounces of blended whisky
Diet 7 UP
Maraschino cherry
Lemon twist

Fill a glass with ice and add blended whisky. Fill up with diet 7 UP and garnish with a cherry and lemon twist.

Nutritional Facts: Protein: 0   Carbohydrates: 0   Calories: 96

Whisky Cobbler

1 teaspoon Splenda® sweetener
3 ounces club soda
2 ounces blended whisky
Cherry
Orange slice
Lemon slice

Dissolve the Splenda® sweetener in the club soda in an old-fashioned glass with crushed ice. Add the whisky and stir. Garnish with the cherry and the orange and lemon slices.

Nutritional Facts: Protein: 0   Carbohydrates: 0   Calories: 128

Whisky Sour

2 ounces blended whisky
1 ounce lemon juice
$^1/_2$ teaspoon Splenda® sweetener
Cherry

Shake all the ingredients in a shaker with ice and strain into a chilled cocktail glass. Garnish with the cherry.

Nutritional Facts: Protein: 0   Carbohydrates: 2.6   Calories: 136

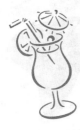

Bourbon Drinks

Admiral Cocktail

1 ounce bourbon
1¹/₂ ounces dry vermouth
¹/₂ ounce lemon juice
Lemon twist

Shake all the ingredients in a shaker with ice and strain into a chilled cocktail glass. Garnish with the lemon twist.

Nutritional Facts: Protein: 0   Carbohydrates: 1.3 grams
Calories: 98

Anchor Splash

1 ounce bourbon
2 teaspoons orange sugar-free syrup
2 teaspoons peach sugar-free syrup
2 teaspoons cherry sugar-free syrup
2 tablespoons heavy cream

Shake all the ingredients into a shaker with ice and strain into an old-fashioned glass with ice.

Nutritional Facts: Protein: 0.6 grams   Carbohydrates: 0.8 grams
Calories: 164

Banana Bird

    1 ounce bourbon
    2 teaspoons banana sugar-free syrup
    2 teaspoons triple sec (substitute orange sugar-free syrup)
    1 ounce heavy cream

Shake all the ingredients in a shaker with ice and strain into a chilled cocktail glass.

Nutritional Facts: Protein: 0.6 grams   Carbohydrates: 0.8 grams
Calories: 164

Blue Grass Cocktail

    1½ ounces bourbon
    1 ounce pineapple juice (substitute pineapple sugar-free
       syrup)
    1 ounce lemon juice
    1 teaspoon cherry sugar-free syrup

Shake all the ingredients in a shaker with ice and strain into a chilled cocktail glass.

Nutritional Facts: Protein: 0   Carbohydrates: 2.6 grams
Calories: 104

Bordever

2 ounces bourbon
1/2 ounce diet ginger ale
Lemon twist

Shake all the ingredients in a shaker with ice and strain into a chilled cocktail glass. Garnish with the lemon twist.

Nutritional Facts: Protein: 0   Carbohydrates: 0   Calories: 128

Bourborita

1 1/2 ounces bourbon
1 1/2 ounces sweet 'n' sour mix (sugar-free)
1/2 ounce triple sec (substitute orange sugar-free syrup)
1/2 ounce pineapple juice (substitute pineapple
    sugar-free syrup)

Shake all the ingredients in a shaker with ice and strain into an old-fashioned glass with ice.

Nutritional Facts: Protein: 0   Carbohydrates: 0   Calories: 96

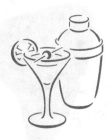

Bourbon Collins

1½ ounces bourbon
½ ounce Rose's Lime Juice
1 teaspoon simple syrup (sugar-free)
Splash of club soda
Lime peel

Mix the bourbon, lime juice, and simple syrup (sugar-free) in a shaker with crushed ice. Pour the mixture into a chilled 12-ounce glass and top off with club soda. Twist the lime peel into the glass and drop in.

Nutritional Facts: Protein: 0   Carbohydrates: 1.4 grams
Calories: 100

Bourbon Daisy

1½ ounces bourbon
½ ounce lemon juice
1 teaspoon cherry sugar-free syrup
Splash of club soda
Orange slice
Pineapple stick

Mix the bourbon, lemon juice and cherry sugar-free syrup in a shaker with crushed ice. Pour into a chilled glass and top off with club soda. Garnish with fruit and serve.

Nutritional Facts: Protein: 0   Carbohydrates: 1.3 grams
Calories: 100

Bourbon Manhattan

> 2 ounces bourbon
> 1/2 ounce red vermouth
> Dash of bitters
> Maraschino cherry

Shake all the ingredients into a shaker with ice and strain into a chilled cocktail glass. Garnish with the cherry.

Nutritional Facts: Protein: 0   Carbohydrates: 0   Calories: 138

Bourbon Eggnog

> 2 ounces bourbon
> 4 ounces half & half
> 1 teaspoon Splenda® sweetener
> 1 ounce eggnog sugar-free syrup
> Grated nutmeg

Shake all the ingredients into a shaker with ice and strain into an old-fashioned glass with ice. Sprinkle the nutmeg on top.

Nutritional Facts: Protein: 4 grams   Carbohydrates: 5 grams
Calories: 268

Bourbon Sour

    2 ounces bourbon
    Juice of $1/2$ lemon
    $1/2$ teaspoon Splenda® sweetener
    Orange slice

Shake all the ingredients in a shaker with ice and strain into an old-fashioned glass with ice. Garnish with the orange slice.

Nutritional Facts: Protein: 0   Carbohydrates: 1.3 grams
Calories: 132

Bourbon Cooler

    3 ounces bourbon
    $1/2$ ounce cherry sugar-free syrup
    Several dashes of peppermint sugar-free syrup
    Several dashes of triple sec (substitute orange
        sugar-free syrup)
    Club soda
    Maraschino cherry
    Orange slice

Mix ingredients in a shaker. Pour into a chilled glass and top off with club soda. Garnish with the cherry and orange slice.

Nutritional Facts: Protein: 0   Carbohydrates: 0   Calories: 192

BOURBON DRINKS

Bourbon Milk Punch

1½ ounces bourbon
4 ounces half & half
1 teaspoon of simple syrup (sugar-free)
Dash of vanilla sugar-free syrup
Grated nutmeg

Shake all the ingredients in a shaker with ice and strain into an old-fashioned glass with ice. Sprinkle with nutmeg.

Nutritional Facts: Protein: 4 grams   Carbohydrates: 5 grams
Calories: 201

Bourbon Orange

1½ ounces bourbon
½ ounce triple sec (substitute orange sugar-free syrup)
1 ounce orange juice (substitute Sugar-Free Tang® for orange juice)
Lemon peel

Shake all the ingredients in a shaker with ice and strain into an old-fashioned glass with ice. Twist the lemon peel into the drink and drop in.

Nutritional Facts: Protein: 0   Carbohydrates: 0   Calories: 96

Bourbon Sidecar

1½ ounces bourbon
¾ ounce triple sec (substitute orange sugar-free syrup)
½ ounce lemon juice

Shake all the ingredients in a shaker with ice and strain into a chilled cocktail glass.

Nutritional Facts: Protein: 0   Carbohydrates: 1.3 grams
Calories: 100

Campfire Sally

1½ ounces bourbon
½ ounce Rose's Lime Juice
½ ounce triple sec (substitute orange sugar-free syrup)

Shake all the ingredients in a shaker with ice and strain into an old-fashioned glass with ice.

Nutritional Facts: Protein: 0   Carbohydrates: 2.8 grams
Calories: 104

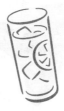

Classic Mint Julep

   6 small mint leaves
   2 ounces bourbon
   1 ounce lemon juice
   1 ounce simple syrup (sugar-free)
   Mint sprig

Crush the mint leaves with the bourbon, lemon juice, and simple syrup in a glass. Add the mixture to a blender with crushed ice. Mix at high speed until the ice becomes mushy. Pour into a chilled double old-fashioned glass and garnish with the mint sprig.

Nutritional Facts: Protein: 0   Carbohydrates: 2.6 grams
Calories: 104

Dan'l Boone

   1½ ounces bourbon
   ½ ounce triple sec (substitute orange sugar-free syrup)
   3 ounces grapefruit juice (substitute Crystal Light® Ruby Red Grapefruit)

Shake all the ingredients in a shaker with ice and strain into an old-fashioned glass with ice.

Nutritional Facts: Protein: 0   Carbohydrates: 0   Calories: 96

Flintstone

 1½ ounces bourbon
 ½ ounce green apple sugar-free syrup
 1 teaspoon lemon juice
 Several dashes of cherry sugar-free syrup
 Several dashes of peppermint sugar-free syrup

Shake all the ingredients in a shaker with ice and strain into a chilled cocktail glass.

Nutritional Facts: Protein: 0   Carbohydrates: 0.7 grams
Calories: 100

Forester

 1 ounce bourbon
 ¾ ounce cherry sugar-free syrup
 1 teaspoon lemon juice
 Maraschino cherry

Shake all the ingredients in a shaker with ice and strain into an old-fashioned glass with ice. Garnish with the cherry.

Nutritional Facts: Protein: 0   Carbohydrates: 0.7 grams
Calories: 66

Golden Boy

1½ ounces bourbon

½ ounce rum

2 ounces orange juice (substitute Sugar-Free Tang® for orange juice)

1 teaspoon lemon juice

Simple syrup (sugar-free)

Shake all the ingredients in a shaker with ice and strain into a chilled cocktail glass.

Nutritional Facts: Protein: 0   Carbohydrates: 0.7 grams Calories: 130.5

Ground Zero

³/₄ ounce bourbon

³/₄ ounce vodka

³/₄ ounce peppermint sugar-free syrup

½ ounce coffee or Kahlua® sugar-free syrup

Shake all the ingredients in a shaker with ice and strain into an old-fashioned glass with ice.

Nutritional Facts: Protein: 0   Carbohydrates: 0   Calories: 97

Home Run

1 ounce bourbon
1 ounce light rum
1 ounce brandy
2 teaspoons lemon juice
Simple syrup (sugar-free) to taste

Shake all the ingredients in a shaker with ice and strain into a chilled cocktail glass.

Nutritional Facts: Protein: 0   Carbohydrates: 1.3 grams
Calories: 204

Imperial

1¹/₂ ounces bourbon
1¹/₂ ounces orange juice (substitute Sugar-Free Tang® for orange juice)
Splash simple syrup (sugar-free)
Splash of club soda

Shake all the ingredients in a shaker with ice and strain into an old-fashioned glass with ice. Top off with club soda.

Nutritional Facts: Protein: 0   Carbohydrates: 0   Calories: 96

BOURBON DRINKS

Julep Mist

1½ ounces bourbon
½ ounce crème de menthe sugar-free syrup
Mint leaf

Shake all the ingredients in a shaker with ice and strain into a cocktail glass filled with crushed ice. Garnish with the mint leaf.

Nutritional Facts: Protein: 0   Carbohydrates: 0   Calories: 96

Kentucky Cappuccino

1 ounce bourbon
1 ounce coffee or Kahlua® sugar-free syrup
4 ounces heavy cream
1 teaspoon instant coffee
2 ounces club soda
Whipped cream
Dark chocolate shavings (CarboRite® sugar-free dark
    chocolate bar)

Mix ingredients in a blender. Pour into a wineglass with ice. Top with whipped cream and garnish with CarboRite® sugar-free dark chocolate bar shavings.

Nutritional Facts: Protein: 2.4 grams   Carbohydrates: 1.6 grams
Calories: 464

Kentucky Cooler

1$\frac{1}{2}$ ounces bourbon
$\frac{1}{2}$ ounce rum
$\frac{1}{4}$ ounce orange juice (substitute Sugar-Free Tang® for
    orange juice)
$\frac{1}{4}$ ounce lemon juice
Dash of cherry sugar-free syrup

Shake all the ingredients in a shaker with ice and strain into a chilled cocktail glass.

Nutritional Facts: Protein: 0   Carbohydrates: 1.3 grams
Calories: 132.5

Kentucky Orange Blossom

1$\frac{1}{2}$ ounces bourbon
$\frac{1}{2}$ ounce of triple sec (substitute orange sugar-free syrup)
1 ounce orange juice (substitute Sugar-Free Tang® for orange
    juice)
Lemon twist

Shake all the ingredients in a shaker with ice and strain into an old-fashioned glass with ice. Garnish with the lemon twist.

Nutritional Facts: Protein: 0   Carbohydrates: 0   Calories: 96

Kentucky Sunrise

1¹/₂ ounces bourbon

3 ounces orange juice (substitute Sugar-Free Tang® for orange juice)

1 teaspoon cherry sugar-free syrup

Pour the bourbon into an old-fashioned glass filled with ice. Add the orange juice and stir. Add the cherry syrup, but do not stir.

Nutritional Facts: Protein: 0   Carbohydrates: 0   Calories: 96

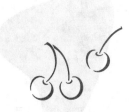

Liquid Love

1 ounce bourbon

¹/₂ ounce lemon juice

Splash of cherry sugar-free syrup

Shake all the ingredients in a shaker with ice and strain into a chilled cocktail glass.

Nutritional Facts: Protein: 0   Carbohydrates: 2.8 grams
Calories: 72

Miami Beach

    1½ ounces bourbon

    1 ounce orange juice (substitute Sugar-Free Tang® for
       orange juice)

    1 ounce pineapple juice (substitute pineapple sugar-free
       syrup)

    1 teaspoon lemon juice

    Several dashes of bitters

    Simple syrup (sugar-free) to taste

Shake all the ingredients in a shaker with ice and strain into an old-fashioned glass with ice.

Nutritional Facts: Protein: 0   Carbohydrates: 0.7 grams
Calories: 98

Peppermint Patty

    1½ ounces bourbon

    ½ ounce peppermint schnapps (substitute peppermint
       sugar-free syrup)

    1 tablespoon lemon juice

    1 teaspoon simple syrup (sugar-free)

    Mint sprig

    Maraschino cherry

Shake all the ingredients in a shaker with ice and strain into an old-fashioned glass with ice. Garnish with the mint sprig and cherry.

Nutritional Facts: Protein: 0   Carbohydrates: 0.7 grams
Calories: 98

Polo Dream

2 ounces bourbon

1 ounce orange juice (substitute Sugar-Free Tang® for orange juice)

3/4 ounce orgeat (substitute almond sugar-free syrup)

Shake all the ingredients in a shaker with ice and strain into a chilled cocktail glass.

Nutritional Facts: Protein: 0   Carbohydrates: 0   Calories: 128

Presbyterian

2 ounces bourbon

Diet ginger ale

Club soda

Pour the bourbon into an old-fashioned glass with ice. Top off the glass with equal parts of the diet ginger ale and club soda.

Nutritional Facts: Protein: 0   Carbohydrates: 0   Calories: 128

Rebel Ringer

1 ounce bourbon

1 ounce crème de menthe (substitute crème de menthe sugar-free syrup)

1 lemon twist

Shake all the ingredients in a shaker with ice and strain into a chilled cocktail glass. Garnish with the lemon twist.

Nutritional Facts: Protein: 0   Carbohydrates: 0   Calories: 64

Rhett Butler Slush

    1¹/₂ ounces bourbon
    1 teaspoon triple sec (substitute orange sugar-free syrup)
    Juice of ¹/₂ lime
    Juice of ¹/₄ lemon
    ¹/₂ teaspoon Splenda® sweetener

Blend all the ingredients in a blender with ice until smooth. Pour into a chilled champagne glass.

Nutritional Facts: Protein: 0   Carbohydrates: 2 grams
Calories: 100

Shanty Hogan

    2 ounces bourbon
    1 ounce simple syrup (sugar-free)
    1 ounce lemon juice
    Maraschino cherry
    6 mint leaves

Blend the ingredients in a blender until smooth. Pour into a glass and garnish with the cherry and mint leaves.

Nutritional Facts: Protein: 0   Carbohydrates: 2.6 grams
Calories: 104

Skyscraper

  2 ounces bourbon
  1 teaspoon Splenda® sweetener
  1 tablespoon lime juice
  Dash of bitters
  3 ounces cranberry juice (Ocean Spray® Light Cranberry Juice
     Cocktail)

Mix the first four ingredients in a shaker and strain into an old-fashioned glass with ice. Top off the glass with the cranberry juice.

Nutritional Facts: Protein: 0   Carbohydrates: 9.8 grams
Calories: 115

Snowman

  3 ounces bourbon
  1 ounce cranberry juice (Ocean Spray® Light Cranberry Juice
     Cocktail)
  1 tablespoon lemon juice
  2 tablespoons simple syrup (sugar-free)

Blend all the ingredients with ice in a blender until smooth. Pour into a chilled wineglass.

Nutritional Facts: Protein: 0   Carbohydrates: 4.2 grams
Calories: 201

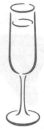

Southern Ginger

1¹/₂ ounces bourbon
1 teaspoon lemon juice
Diet ginger ale
Lemon twist

Mix the first two ingredients in a shaker and pour into an old-fashioned glass with ice. Top off with the diet ginger ale. Twist the lemon peel and drop it in the drink.

Nutritional Facts: Protein: 0   Carbohydrates: 0.7 grams
Calories: 98

Spinner

1¹/₂ ounces bourbon
1 ounce orange juice (substitute Sugar-Free Tang® for orange juice)
1 tablespoon lime juice
1 teaspoon Splenda® sweetener
¹/₂ orange slice

Shake all the ingredients in a shaker with ice and strain into an old-fashioned glass with ice. Garnish with the orange slice.

Nutritional Facts: Protein: 0   Carbohydrates: 1.4 grams
Calories: 100

Stone Sour

    1¹/₂ ounces bourbon
    ¹/₂ ounce lemon juice
    1 teaspoon crème de menthe (substitute crème de menthe
        sugar-free syrup)
    1 teaspoon Splenda® sweetener
    Club soda

Fill a glass with crushed ice. Pour in bourbon, lemon juice, crème de menthe and Splenda® sweetener. Stir and top off with club soda.

Nutritional Facts: Protein: 0   Carbohydrates: 1.3 grams
Calories: 100

Sweet and Sour Bourbon

    1¹/₂ ounces bourbon
    4 ounces orange juice (substitute Sugar-Free Tang® for
        orange juice)
    1 or 2 pinches of Splenda® sweetener
    1 pinch of salt
    Maraschino cherry

Shake all the ingredients in a shaker with ice and strain into an old-fashioned glass with ice. Garnish with the cherry.

Nutritional Facts: Protein: 0   Carbohydrates: 0   Calories: 96

Trolley

 2 ounces bourbon
 Cranberry juice (Ocean Spray® Light Cranberry Juice Cocktail)
 Pineapple juice (substitute Crystal Light® Pineapple Orange)

Fill an old-fashioned glass with ice and add bourbon. Fill with equal parts of cranberry and pineapple juice and stir.

Nutritional Facts: Protein: 0   Carbohydrates: 2.8 grams
Calories: 133

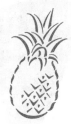

Ward Eight

 2 ounces bourbon
 1 ounce lemon juice
 1 ounce orange juice (substitute Sugar-Free Tang® for orange juice)
 Simple syrup (sugar-free) to taste
 Dash of grenadine (substitute cherry sugar-free syrup)

Shake all the ingredients in a shaker with ice and strain into a chilled cocktail glass.

Nutritional Facts: Protein: 0   Carbohydrates: 2.6 grams
Calories: 136

BOURBON DRINKS

Brandy Drinks

American Beauty

>   ³/₄ ounce brandy
>   ³/₄ ounce dry vermouth
>   ¹/₂ ounce grenadine (substitute cherry sugar-free syrup)
>   ³/₄ ounce orange juice (substitute Sugar-Free Tang® for
>   orange juice)
>   ¹/₂ ounce crème de menthe (substitute crème de menthe
>   sugar-free syrup)

Shake all the ingredients in a shaker with ice and strain into a chilled cocktail glass.

Nutritional Facts: Protein: 0   Carbohydrates: 0   Calories: 80

Apple Blossom

>   1¹/₂ ounces brandy
>   1 ounce green apple sugar-free syrup
>   1 teaspoon lemon juice
>   Lemon slice

Shake all the ingredients in a shaker with ice and strain into a chilled cocktail glass. Garnish with the lemon slice.

Nutritional Facts: Protein: 0   Carbohydrates: 0.7 grams
Calories: 108.5

Banana Peel

1½ ounces brandy
¾ ounce banana sugar-free syrup
1 ounce heavy cream
½ ounce lemon juice
Club soda
Lemon wedge

Mix the ingredients in a shaker. Pour the mixture into an old-fashioned glass with ice and top off with the club soda. Stir gently and garnish with the lemon wedge.

Nutritional Facts: Protein: 0.6 grams   Carbohydrates: 1.7 grams
Calories: 208.5

Beau's Sister

1½ ounces brandy
1 ounce crème de menthe (substitute crème de menthe sugar-free syrup)
1 ounce heavy cream

Shake all the ingredients in a shaker with ice and strain into a chilled cocktail glass.

Nutritional Facts: Protein: 0.6 grams   Carbohydrates: 0.4 grams
Calories: 206.5

Brandy Daisy

   2 ounces brandy

   1 ounce lemon juice

   ½ teaspoon Splenda® sweetener

   ½ ounce grenadine (substitute cherry sugar-free syrup)

Shake all the ingredients in a shaker with ice and strain into a chilled cocktail glass.

Nutritional Facts: Protein: 0   Carbohydrates: 2.6 grams
Calories: 150

Between the Sheets

   1 ounce brandy

   ¾ ounce triple sec (substitute orange sugar-free syrup)

   1 ounce light rum

   ¾ ounce sweet 'n' sour mix (sugar-free)

Shake all the ingredients in a shaker with ice and strain into an old-fashioned glass with ice.

Nutritional Facts: Protein: 0   Carbohydrates: 0   Calories: 136

Brandy Eggnog

    2 ounces brandy
    1 ounce eggnog sugar-free syrup
    6 ounces half & half
    Ground nutmeg

Shake all the ingredients in a shaker with ice and strain into an old-fashioned glass with ice. Sprinkle with nutmeg.

Nutritional Facts: Protein: 6 grams   Carbohydrates: 7 grams
Calories: 562

Brandy Fix

    2 ounces brandy
    1 ounce lemon juice
    1 ounce water
    1 teaspoon Splenda® sweetener
    Cherry
    Lemon slice

Shake all the ingredients in a shaker with ice and strain into an old-fashioned glass with ice. Garnish with the cherry and lemon slice.

Nutritional Facts: Protein: 0   Carbohydrates: 2.6 grams
Calories: 150

Brandy Fizz

- 2 ounces brandy
- 4 ounces club soda
- 1 ounce lemon juice
- 1 teaspoon Splenda® sweetener

Shake all the ingredients in a shaker with ice and strain into an old-fashioned glass with ice.

Nutritional Facts: Protein: 0   Carbohydrates: 2.6 grams
Calories: 150

Brandy Highball

- 2 ounces brandy
- Club soda
- Lemon twist

Mix both the ingredients in a glass over crushed ice and stir. Garnish with a lemon twist.

Nutritional Facts: Protein: 0   Carbohydrates: 0   Calories: 142

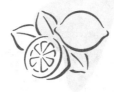

Brandy Julep

  2 ounces brandy
  1 teaspoon Splenda® sweetener
  Cherry
  4 mint leaves

Shake all the ingredients in a shaker with ice and strain into an old-fashioned glass with ice. Garnish with the cherry and mint leaves.

Nutritional Facts: Protein: 0   Carbohydrates: 0   Calories: 142

Brandy Manhattan

  2 ounces brandy
  ¹/₂ ounce sweet or dry vermouth
  Dash of bitters
  Maraschino cherry

Shake all the ingredients in a shaker with ice and strain into a chilled cocktail glass. Garnish with the cherry.

Nutritional Facts: Protein: 0   Carbohydrates: 0   Calories: 182

Brandy Old-Fashioned

    1 teaspoon Splenda® sweetener
    Several dashes of bitters
    3 ounces brandy
    Lemon peel

Place the Splenda® sweetener in a chilled old-fashioned glass. Add the bitters and a dash of cold water to dissolve the sweetener. Add ice cubes and the brandy. Twist the lemon peel over the drink and drop in.

Nutritional Facts: Protein: 0   Carbohydrates: 0   Calories: 213

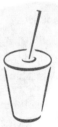

Brandy Milk Punch

    2 ounces brandy
    4 ounces half & half
    1 teaspoon Splenda® sweetener
    ¼ teaspoon nutmeg

Shake all the ingredients in a shaker with ice and strain into an old-fashioned glass with ice. Garnish with nutmeg.

Nutritional Facts: Protein: 4 grams   Carbohydrates: 5 grams Calories: 352

Brandy Sling

  2 ounces brandy
  1 ounce lemon juice
  1 ounce water
  1 teaspoon Splenda® sweetener
  Lemon twist

Shake all the ingredients in a shaker with ice and strain into a chilled cocktail glass. Garnish with a lemon twist.

Nutritional Facts: Protein: 0   Carbohydrates: 2.6 grams
Calories: 180

Brandy Smash

  4 fresh mint sprigs
  1 teaspoon Splenda® sweetener
  1 ounce club soda
  2 ounces brandy
  Cherry
  Orange slice

Crush the mint sprigs with the Splenda® sweetener and club soda in an old-fashioned glass. Add brandy over ice and stir. Garnish with the cherry and orange slice.

Nutritional Facts: Protein: 0   Carbohydrates: 0   Calories: 142

BRANDY DRINKS

Brandy Sour

    2 ounces brandy
    1 ounce lemon juice
    $\frac{1}{2}$ teaspoon Splenda® sweetener
    Cherry
    Orange slice

Shake all the ingredients in a shaker with ice and strain into an old-fashioned glass with ice. Garnish with the cherry and orange slice.

Nutritional Facts: Protein: 0   Carbohydrates: 2.6 grams
Calories: 150

Brandy Swizzle

    2 ounces brandy
    $\frac{1}{2}$ ounce lime juice
    1 teaspoon Splenda® sweetener
    1 dash of bitters
    3 ounces club soda

Shake the brandy, lime juice, Splenda® sweetener, and bitters in a shaker with ice and strain into an old-fashioned glass with ice. Add the club soda and stir. Serve with a swizzle stick.

Nutritional Facts: Protein: 0   Carbohydrates: 1.4 grams
Calories: 146

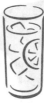

Charles Cocktail

- 2 ounces brandy
- $1/2$ ounce sweet vermouth
- 2 dashes of bitters

Shake all the ingredients in a shaker with ice and strain into a chilled cocktail glass.

Nutritional Facts: Protein: 0   Carbohydrates: 0   Calories: 152

Cherry Blossom

- 2 ounces brandy
- 1 ounce cherry sugar-free syrup
- $1/2$ ounce lemon juice
- 1 ounce triple sec (substitute orange sugar-free syrup)
- Cherry

Shake all the ingredients in a shaker with ice and strain into a chilled cocktail glass. Garnish with the cherry.

Nutritional Facts: Protein: 0   Carbohydrates: 1.3 grams
Calories: 146

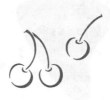

Fancy Brandy

2 ounces brandy

$\frac{1}{3}$ teaspoon Splenda® sweetener

$\frac{1}{2}$ teaspoon triple sec (substitute with orange sugar-free syrup)

2 dashes of bitters

Lemon twist

Shake all the ingredients in a shaker with ice and strain into a chilled cocktail glass. Garnish with the lemon twist.

Nutritional Facts: Protein: 0   Carbohydrates: 0   Calories: 142

Harvard Cocktail

2 ounces brandy

1 ounce sweet vermouth

1 ounce lemon juice

1 teaspoon grenadine (substitute cherry sugar-free syrup)

1 dash of bitters

Shake all the ingredients in a shaker with ice and strain into a chilled cocktail glass.

Nutritional Facts: Protein: 0   Carbohydrates: 2.6 grams
Calories: 170

La Jolla

   2 ounces brandy
   $^{1}/_{2}$ ounce lemon juice
   1 teaspoon orgeat (substitute almond sugar-free syrup)
   1 dash of bitters
   Lemon twist

Shake all the ingredients in a shaker with ice and strain into a chilled cocktail glass. Garnish with the lemon twist.

Nutritional Facts: Protein: 0   Carbohydrates: 1.3 grams
Calories: 176

Sidecar

   2 ounces brandy
   1 ounce lemon juice
   1 ounce triple sec (substitute orange sugar-free syrup)

Shake all the ingredients in a shaker with ice and strain into a chilled cocktail glass.

Nutritional Facts: Protein: 0   Carbohydrates: 2.6 grams
Calories: 150

BRANDY DRINKS

Stinger

2 ounces brandy
½ ounce crème de menthe sugar-free syrup

Shake all the ingredients in a shaker with ice and strain into a chilled cocktail glass.

Nutritional Facts: Protein: 0   Carbohydrates: 0   Calories: 142

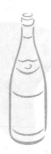

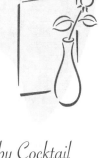

Gin Drinks

Abby Cocktail

2 ounces gin
1¹/₂ ounces orange juice (substitute Sugar-Free Tang® for
    orange juice)
2 dashes of bitters
Cherry

Shake all the ingredients in a shaker with ice and strain into a chilled cocktail glass. Garnish with a cherry.

Nutritional Facts: Protein: 0   Carbohydrates: 0   Calories: 130

Artillery

2 ounces gin
1 ounce sweet vermouth
2 dashes of bitters

Shake all the ingredients in a shaker with ice and strain into a chilled cocktail glass.

Nutritional Facts: Protein: 0   Carbohydrates: 0   Calories: 140

Bennet Cocktail

> 2 ounces gin
> 1 ounce lime juice
> 1 teaspoon Splenda® sweetener
> 2 dashes of orange bitters

Shake all the ingredients in a shaker with ice and strain into a chilled cocktail glass.

Nutritional Facts: Protein: 0   Carbohydrates: 2.8 grams
Calories: 138

Boomerang

> 2 ounces gin
> 1 ounce dry vermouth
> ¹/₂ ounce cherry sugar-free syrup
> 2 dashes of bitters
> Cherry

Shake all the ingredients in a shaker with ice and strain into a chilled cocktail glass. Garnish with the cherry.

Nutritional Facts: Protein: 0   Carbohydrates: 0   Calories: 140

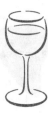

Bronx Cocktail

2 ounces gin
¹/₂ ounce orange juice (substitute Sugar-Free Tang® for orange juice)
¹/₂ ounce dry vermouth
¹/₂ ounce sweet vermouth

Shake all the ingredients in a shaker with ice and strain into a chilled cocktail glass.

Nutritional Facts: Protein: 0   Carbohydrates: 0   Calories: 150

Caruso

2 ounces gin
1 ounce dry vermouth
1 ounce crème de menthe sugar-free syrup

Shake all the ingredients in a shaker with ice and strain into a cocktail glass.

Nutritional Facts: Protein: 0   Carbohydrates: 0   Calories: 150

Casino

    2 ounces gin
    1 ounce lemon juice
    1 teaspoon cherry sugar-free syrup
    2 dashes of bitters

Shake all the ingredients in a shaker with ice and strain into a chilled cocktail glass.

Nutritional Facts: Protein: 0   Carbohydrates: 2.6 grams
Calories: 138

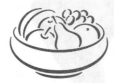

Chelsea Hotel

    2 ounces gin
    1 ounce triple sec (substitute orange sugar-free syrup)
    1 ounce lemon juice

Shake all the ingredients in a shaker with ice and strain into a chilled cocktail glass.

Nutritional Facts: Protein: 0   Carbohydrates: 2.6 grams
Calories: 138

Delmonico

    1 ounce gin
    $^1/_2$ ounce brandy
    $^1/_2$ ounce sweet vermouth
    $^1/_2$ ounce dry vermouth
    1 dash of bitters
    Lemon peel

Shake all the ingredients in a shaker with ice and strain into a chilled cocktail glass. Garnish with the lemon peel.

Nutritional Facts: Protein: 0   Carbohydrates: 0   Calories: 120.5

Emerald Isle

    2 ounces gin
    1 teaspoon crème de menthe sugar-free syrup
    2 dashes of bitters

Shake all the ingredients in a shaker with ice and strain into a chilled cocktail glass.

Nutritional Facts: Protein: 0   Carbohydrates: 0   Calories: 130

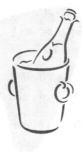

GIN DRINKS

Emerson

2 ounces gin
1 ounce sweet vermouth
½ ounce lemon juice
½ ounce cherry sugar-free syrup

Shake all the ingredients in a shaker with ice and strain into a chilled cocktail glass.

Nutritional Facts: Protein: 0   Carbohydrates: 2.6 grams
Calories: 154

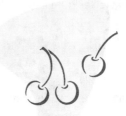

Farmer's Cocktail

2 ounces gin
1 ounce dry vermouth
1 ounce sweet vermouth
2 dashes of bitters
Lemon twist

Shake all the ingredients in a shaker with ice and strain into a chilled cocktail glass. Garnish with the lemon twist.

Nutritional Facts: Protein: 0   Carbohydrates: 0   Calories: 170

Fifty-Fifty

   2 ounces gin
   2 ounces dry vermouth
   Cocktail olive

Shake all the ingredients in a shaker with ice and strain into a chilled cocktail glass. Garnish with the cocktail olive.

Nutritional Facts: Protein: 0   Carbohydrates: 0   Calories: 170

Gin Gimlet

   2 ounces gin
   1 ounce Rose's Lime Juice
   Lime wedge

Shake both the ingredients in a shaker with ice and strain into a chilled cocktail glass. Garnish with the lime wedge.

Nutritional Facts: Protein: 0   Carbohydrates: 2.8 grams
Calories: 138

Gin and Sin

> 2 ounces gin
> 1 ounce lemon juice
> 1 ounce orange juice (substitute Sugar-Free Tang® for orange juice)
> ½ teaspoon grenadine (substitute cherry sugar-free syrup)

Shake all the ingredients in a shaker with ice and strain into a chilled cocktail glass.

Nutritional Facts: Protein: 0   Carbohydrates: 2.6 grams   Calories: 138

Gin and Tonic

> 2 ounces gin
> 5 ounces diet tonic water
> Lime wedge

Shake both the ingredients in a shaker with ice and strain into an old-fashioned glass with ice. Garnish with the lime wedge.

Nutritional Facts: Protein: 0   Carbohydrates: 0   Calories: 130

Gin Cobbler

> 1 teaspoon Splenda® sweetener
> 3 ounces club soda
> 2 ounces gin
> Cherry
> Orange slice
> Lemon slice

Dissolve the Splenda® sweetener in the club soda in an old-fashioned glass with crushed ice. Add the gin and stir. Garnish with the fruits.

Nutritional Facts: Protein: 0   Carbohydrates: 0   Calories: 130

Gin Cooler

> 2 ounces gin
> 4 ounces diet lemon-lime soda
> Lemon wedge

Mix the gin and diet lemon-lime soda in an old-fashioned glass with ice and stir. Garnish with the lemon wedge.

Nutritional Facts: Protein: 0   Carbohydrates: 0   Calories: 130

Gin Daisy

2 ounces gin
1 ounce lemon juice
1 teaspoon grenadine (substitute cherry sugar-free syrup)
$\frac{1}{2}$ teaspoon Splenda® sweetener
Cherry
Orange slice

Shake all the ingredients in a shaker with ice and strain into an old-fashioned glass over crushed ice. Garnish with the fruits.

Nutritional Facts: Protein: 0   Carbohydrates: 2.6 grams
Calories: 138

Gin Fix

1 ounce lemon juice
1 teaspoon Splenda® sweetener
2 teaspoons water
2 ounces gin
Cherry

Shake all the ingredients except the gin in a shaker with ice and strain into an old-fashioned glass over crushed ice. Pour the gin on top and stir. Garnish with the cherry.

Nutritional Facts: Protein: 0   Carbohydrates: 2.6 grams
Calories: 138

Gin Martini

2 ounces gin
1 teaspoon dry vermouth
Cocktail olive
Cocktail onion (optional)

Shake all the ingredients in a shaker with ice and strain into a chilled cocktail glass. Garnish with the cocktail olive and onion.

Nutritional Facts: Protein: 0   Carbohydrates: 0   Calories: 135

Gin Milk Punch

2 ounces gin
4 ounces half & half
1 teaspoon Splenda® sweetener
$1/4$ teaspoon nutmeg

Shake all the ingredients in a shaker with ice and strain into a chilled cocktail glass over crushed ice. Garnish with nutmeg.

Nutritional Facts: Protein: 4 grams   Carbohydrates: 5 grams
Calories: 280

Gin Sling

>   2 ounces gin
>   2 ounces lemon juice
>   1 teaspoon Splenda® sweetener
>   2 teaspoons water
>   Lemon twist

Shake all the ingredients in a shaker with ice and strain into an old-fashioned glass with ice. Garnish with the lemon twist.

Nutritional Facts: Protein: 0   Carbohydrates: 5.2 grams
Calories: 146

Gin Smash

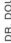

>   1 teaspoon Splenda® sweetener
>   4 fresh mint sprigs
>   1 ounce club soda
>   2 ounces gin
>   Lemon twist

Crush the Splenda® sweetener with the mint sprigs and club soda in an old-fashioned glass. Add the gin over ice and stir. Garnish with the lemon twist.

Nutritional Facts: Protein: 0   Carbohydrates: 0   Calories: 130

Gin Sour

2 ounces gin
1 ounce lemon juice
½ teaspoon Splenda® sweetener
Cherry

Shake all the ingredients in a shaker with ice and strain into an old-fashioned glass with ice. Garnish with the cherry.

Nutritional Facts: Protein: 0   Carbohydrates: 2.6 grams
Calories: 138

Gin Swizzle

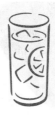

2 ounces gin
1 ounce Rose's Lime Juice
1 teaspoon Splenda® sweetener
2 dashes of bitters
2 ounces club soda

Mix the gin, lime juice, Splenda® sweetener and bitters in a shaker with ice. Strain into an old-fashioned glass over crushed ice. Add the club soda and stir.

Nutritional Facts: Protein: 0   Carbohydrates: 2.8 grams
Calories: 138

Harlem Cocktail

2 ounces gin
½ ounce pineapple sugar-free syrup
½ ounce cherry sugar-free syrup

Shake all the ingredients in a shaker with ice and strain into a chilled cocktail glass.

Nutritional Facts: Protein: 0   Carbohydrates: 0   Calories: 130

Hawaiian Cocktail

2 ounces gin
½ ounce pineapple sugar-free syrup
½ ounce triple sec (substitute orange sugar-free syrup)
Cherry

Shake all the ingredients in a shaker with ice and strain into a chilled cocktail glass. Garnish with the cherry.

Nutritional Facts: Protein: 0   Carbohydrates: 0   Calories: 130

Honolulu Cocktail

- 2 ounces gin
- $^1/_2$ ounce sugar-free pineapple syrup
- $^1/_2$ ounce lemon juice
- $^1/_2$ ounce Rose's Lime Juice
- $^1/_2$ ounce orange juice (substitute Sugar-Free Tang® for orange juice)
- $^1/_2$ teaspoon Splenda® sweetener

Shake all the ingredients in a shaker with ice and strain into a chilled cocktail glass.

Nutritional Facts: Protein: 0   Carbohydrates: 2.7 grams
Calories: 138

Hula Hoop

- 2 ounces gin
- 1 ounce orange juice (substitute Sugar-Free Tang® for orange juice)
- $^1/_2$ ounce sugar-free pineapple syrup
- Cherry

Shake all the ingredients in a shaker with ice and strain into a chilled cocktail glass. Garnish with the cherry.

Nutritional Facts: Protein: 0   Carbohydrates: 0   Calories: 130

GIN DRINKS

Melon Ball

    $1\frac{1}{2}$ ounces gin
    $\frac{1}{2}$ ounce sugar-free watermelon syrup
    $\frac{1}{2}$ ounce triple sec (substitute orange sugar-free syrup)
    $\frac{1}{2}$ ounce lemon juice

Shake all the ingredients in a shaker with ice and strain into a chilled cocktail glass.

Nutritional Facts: Protein: 0   Carbohydrates: 1.3 grams
Calories: 101.5

Opal Cocktail

    2 ounces gin
    1 ounce orange juice (substitute Sugar-Free Tang® for
        orange juice)
    $\frac{1}{2}$ ounce triple sec (substitute orange sugar-free syrup)
    $\frac{1}{2}$ teaspoon Splenda® sweetener

Shake all the ingredients in a shaker with ice and strain into a chilled cocktail glass.

Nutritional Facts: Protein: 0   Carbohydrates: 0   Calories: 130

Orange Blossom

- 2 ounces gin
- 1 ounce orange juice (substitute Sugar-Free Tang® for orange juice)
- 1 teaspoon Splenda® sweetener
- Orange slice

Shake all the ingredients in a shaker with ice and strain into a chilled cocktail glass. Garnish with the orange slice.

Nutritional Facts: Protein: 0   Carbohydrates: 0   Calories: 130

Princeton Cocktail

- 1 ounce gin
- 1 ounce dry vermouth
- 1 ounce Rose's Lime Juice

Shake all the ingredients in a shaker with ice and strain into a chilled cocktail glass.

Nutritional Facts: Protein: 0   Carbohydrates: 2.8 grams Calories: 93

Vodka Drinks

Belmont Stakes

1¹/₂ ounces vodka

¹/₂ ounce gold rum

¹/₂ ounce strawberry sugar-free syrup

¹/₂ ounce Rose's Lime Juice

¹/₂ teaspoon grenadine (substitute cherry sugar-free syrup)

1 orange slice

Shake all the ingredients in a shaker with ice and strain into a chilled cocktail glass. Garnish with the orange slice.

Nutritional Facts: Protein: 0   Carbohydrates: 1.4 grams
Calories: 134

Bull Shot

2 ounces vodka
4 ounces beef bouillon
Several dashes Tabasco sauce
Black pepper
Salt
Several dashes of Worcestershire sauce
1 teaspoon lemon juice
$^1/_2$ teaspoon horseradish
Pinch of celery salt

Shake all the ingredients in a shaker with ice and strain into an old-fashioned glass with ice.

Nutritional Facts: Protein: 1.2 grams   Carbohydrates: 0.7 grams
Calories: 132

Cape Codder

2 ounces vodka
Dash of Rose's Lime Juice
2 ounces cranberry juice (Ocean Spray® Light Cranberry Juice Cocktail)
1 teaspoon simple syrup (sugar-free)

Shake all the ingredients in a shaker with ice and strain into a chilled old-fashioned glass with ice.

Nutritional Facts: Protein: 0   Carbohydrates: 5.6 grams
Calories: 140

Chiquita

2 ounces vodka
$^1/_2$ ounce banana sugar-free syrup
$^1/_2$ ounce Rose's Lime Juice
1 teaspoon orgeat (substitute sugar-free almond syrup)

Shake all the ingredients in a shaker with ice and strain into a chilled cocktail glass.

Nutritional Facts: Protein: 0   Carbohydrates: 1.4 grams
Calories: 134

Coffee Cooler

2 ounces vodka
1 ounce coffee or Kahlua® sugar-free syrup
1 ounce heavy cream
4 ounces iced coffee

Shake all the ingredients in a shaker with ice and strain into an old-fashioned glass with ice.

Nutritional Facts: Protein: 1 gram   Carbohydrates: 1 gram
Calories: 230

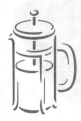

Cosmopolitan

- 2 ounces vodka
- 1/2 ounce triple sec or sugar-free orange syrup
- 1/2 ounce cranberry juice (Ocean Spray® Light Cranberry Juice Cocktail)
- 1/2 ounce Rose's Lime Juice

Shake all the ingredients in a shaker with ice and strain into a chilled cocktail glass.

Nutritional Facts: Protein: 0   Carbohydrates: 2.8 grams
Calories: 134

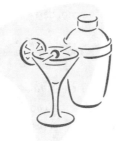

Dr. John's Sugar-Free Lemoncello

15 lemons
2 bottles (750 ml) 40% (80 proof) vodka
108 packets Splenda® no calorie sweetener
4-quart mason jar or similar sealable glass container

Wash the lemons in hot water. Remove the yellow layer of peel with vegetable peeler, being careful to avoid taking any of the white pith of the lemon. If necessary, use a knife to scrape the white pith off the yellow peel. Put the yellow peels in the mason jar and cover with one bottle of vodka. Stir, cover and store the jar in a cool dark place for 40 days and 40 nights.

After 40 days and 40 nights, add the second bottle of vodka to the vodka lemon mix. Add the Splenda® and stir until dissolved. Cover and return the jar to the cool dark place for another 40 days and 40 nights.

After the second 40 days and 40 nights, strain the mixture and discard the lemon peel.

Pour the lemoncello into clean bottles with caps or corks. Store the bottles of lemoncello in a cool pantry or cupboard and store one bottle in the freezer until served.

Serve the ice cold lemoncello in small cordial glasses and enjoy!

Notes: You don't need to use expensive vodka to make lemoncello. A moderate-priced vodka will make very good lemoncello.

Use Splenda® packets rather than granular sweetener because they have less filler and therefore dissolve better.

Nutritional Facts: Protein: 0   Carbohydrates: 0   Calories: 130

Ellen's Lemon Fizz

  2 ounces lemon vodka
  4 ounces diet tonic
  1 lemon wedge

Mix all the ingredients in an old-fashioned glass with ice. Garnish with the lemon wedge.

Nutritional Facts: Protein: 0   Carbohydrates: 0   Calories: 130

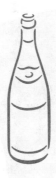

Firefly

  2 ounces vodka
  4 ounces grapefruit juice (substitute Crystal Light® Ruby
    Red Grapefruit)
  1 ounce grenadine (substitute cherry sugar-free syrup)

Shake all the ingredients in a shaker and strain into an old-fashioned glass with ice.

Nutritional Facts: Protein: 0   Carbohydrates: 0   Calories: 130

VODKA DRINKS

Fuzzy Navel

>   2 ounces vodka
>   ½ ounce peach sugar-free syrup
>   6 ounces orange juice (substitute Sugar-Free Tang®
>   for orange juice)
>   Orange slice

Shake all the ingredients in a shaker with ice and strain into an old-fashioned glass with ice. Garnish with the orange.

Nutritional Facts: Protein: 0   Carbohydrates: 0   Calories: 130

Gingersnap

>   3 ounces vodka
>   1 ounce gingerbread sugar-free syrup
>   Club soda

Mix the vodka and gingerbread sugar-free syrup in a shaker with ice and strain into an old-fashioned glass with ice. Top off with the club soda.

Nutritional Facts: Protein: 0   Carbohydrates: 0   Calories: 195

Godmother

>   2 ounces vodka
>   1 ounce amaretto sugar-free syrup

Shake all the ingredients into a shaker with ice and strain into a chilled cocktail glass.

Nutritional Facts: Protein: 0   Carbohydrates: 0   Calories: 130

Green Spider

2 ounces vodka
$\frac{1}{2}$ ounce crème de menthe sugar-free syrup

Shake all the ingredients in a shaker with ice and strain into an old-fashioned glass with ice.

Nutritional Facts: Protein: 0   Carbohydrates: 0   Calories: 130

Ice Pick

$1\frac{1}{2}$ ounces vodka
6 ounces iced tea
1 teaspoon Splenda® sweetener
Lemon wedge

Shake all the ingredients in a shaker with ice and strain into an old-fashioned glass with ice. Garnish with the lemon wedge.

Nutritional Facts: Protein: 0   Carbohydrates: 0   Calories: 97.5

Jungle Joe

2 ounces vodka
$\frac{1}{2}$ ounce banana sugar-free syrup
1 ounce half & half

Shake all the ingredients in a shaker with ice and strain into an old-fashioned glass with ice.

Nutritional Facts: Protein: 1 gram   Carbohydrates: 1 gram
Calories: 230

Kamikaze

> 2 ounces vodka
> 1 teaspoon Rose's Lime Juice
> $^1/_2$ ounce triple sec (substitute orange sugar-free syrup)

Shake all the ingredients in a shaker with ice and strain into a chilled cocktail glass.

Nutritional Facts: Protein: 0   Carbohydrates: 0.7 grams
Calories: 132

Kremlin

> 2 ounces vodka
> 1 ounce coffee or Kahlua® sugar-free syrup
> 1 ounce half & half

Combine all the ingredients in a blender with ice and blend until smooth. Pour into a chilled cocktail glass.

Nutritional Facts: Protein: 1 gram   Carbohydrates: 1 gram
Calories: 230

Lemon Aid

    2 ounces lemon vodka
    4 ounces sweet 'n' sour (sugar-free)
    1 teaspoon Rose's Lime Juice

Shake all the ingredients in a shaker with ice and strain into an old-fashioned glass with ice.

Nutritional Facts: Protein: 0   Carbohydrates: 0.7 grams
Calories: 132

Long Island Iced Tea

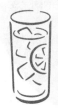

    1 ounce vodka
    1 ounce gin
    1 ounce light rum
    1 ounce tequila
    1 ounce lemon juice
    $\frac{1}{2}$ ounce triple sec (substitute orange sugar-free syrup)
    3 ounces diet cola
    Lime wedge
    Cherry

Shake all the ingredients in a shaker with ice and strain into an old-fashioned glass with ice. Garnish with the lime wedge and cherry.

Nutritional Facts: Protein: 0   Carbohydrates: 2.6 grams
Calories: 268

VODKA DRINKS

Madras

> 2 ounces vodka
>
> 2 ounces orange juice (substitute Sugar-Free Tang® for orange juice)
>
> 1 ounce cranberry juice (Ocean Spray® Light Cranberry Juice Cocktail)

Shake all the ingredients in a shaker with ice and strain into a chilled cocktail glass.

Nutritional Facts: Protein: 0   Carbohydrates: 2.8   Calories: 135

Moscow Milk Toddy

> 1½ ounces vodka
>
> ½ ounce grenadine (substitute cherry sugar-free syrup)
>
> 4 ounces half & half
>
> Powdered cinnamon

Shake all the ingredients in a shaker with ice and strain into an old-fashioned glass with ice. Sprinkle the cinnamon on top.

Nutritional Facts: Protein: 4 grams   Carbohydrates: 5 grams
Calories: 377.5

Polynesian Pepper Pot

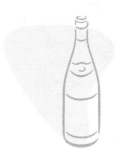

- 1½ ounces vodka
- ¾ ounce gold rum
- 2 ounces pineapple sugar-free syrup
- ½ ounce orgeat (substitute almond sugar-free syrup)
- ½ teaspoon lemon juice
- 1 tablespoon heavy cream
- Several dashes of Tabasco
- ½ teaspoon cayenne pepper
- Curry powder

Shake all the ingredients in a shaker with ice and strain into an old-fashioned glass with ice. Sprinkle the curry powder on top.

Nutritional Facts: Protein: 0.5 grams   Carbohydrates: 0.6 grams
Calories: 212.5

Russian Coffee

- 2 ounces vodka
- 1 ounce coffee or Kahlua® sugar-free syrup
- 1 ounce heavy cream

Mix all the ingredients in a blender with ice. Blend until smooth and pour into a chilled old-fashioned glass.

Nutritional Facts: Protein: 1 gram   Carbohydrates: 1 gram
Calories: 230

VODKA DRINKS

Russian Rose

 2 ounces vodka
 $1/2$ ounce grenadine (substitute cherry sugar-free syrup)
 Dash of bitters

Shake all the ingredients in a shaker with ice and strain into a chilled cocktail glass.

Nutritional Facts: Protein: 0   Carbohydrates: 0   Calories: 130

Salty Dog

 2 ounces vodka
 5 ounces grapefruit juice (substitute Crystal Light® Ruby Red
    Grapefruit for grapefruit juice)
 2 teaspoons salt
 Lime wedge

Shake all the ingredients in a shaker with ice and strain into a chilled cocktail glass. Garnish with the lime wedge.

Nutritional Facts: Protein: 0   Carbohydrates: 0   Calories: 130

Screwdriver

 2 ounces vodka
 4 ounces orange juice (substitute Sugar-Free Tang® for
    orange juice)

Mix the ingredients in an old-fashioned glass with ice.

Nutritional Facts: Protein: 0   Carbohydrates: 0   Calories: 130

Sea Breeze

2 ounces vodka

2 ounces cranberry juice (Ocean Spray® Light Cranberry
Juice Cocktail)

2 ounces grapefruit juice (substitute Crystal Light® Ruby Red
Grapefruit for grapefruit juice)

Lime wedge

Shake all the ingredients in a shaker with ice and strain into an old-
fashioned glass with ice. Garnish with the lime wedge.

Nutritional Facts: Protein: 0   Carbohydrates: 5.6 grams
Calories: 140

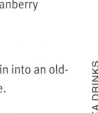

Sex on the Beach

1 ounce vodka

1 ounce peach sugar-free syrup

2 ounces orange juice (substitute Sugar-Free Tang® for
orange juice)

2 ounces cranberry juice (Ocean Spray® Light Cranberry
Juice Cocktail)

Lime wedge

Shake all the ingredients in a shaker with ice and strain into an old-
fashioned glass with ice. Garnish with the lime wedge.

Nutritional Facts: Protein: 0   Carbohydrates: 5.6 grams
Calories: 75

Vodka Cobbler

    1 teaspoon Splenda® sweetener
    3 ounces club soda
    2 ounces vodka
    Cherry
    Orange slice
    Lemon slice

Dissolve the Splenda® sweetener in the club soda in an old-fashioned glass with ice. Add the vodka and stir. Garnish with the cherry and the orange and lemon slices.

Nutritional Facts: Protein: 0   Carbohydrates: 0   Calories: 130

Vodka Cooler

    1^1/$_2$ ounces vodka
    ^{1}/$_2$ ounce sweet vermouth
    ^{1}/$_2$ ounce lemon juice
    ^{1}/$_2$ ounce simple syrup (sugar-free)
    Club soda

Shake all the ingredients in a shaker with ice and strain into an old-fashioned glass with ice. Top off with the club soda.

Nutritional Facts: Protein: 0   Carbohydrates: 1.3 grams Calories: 111.5

Vodka Collins

 2 ounces vodka
 1 ounce lemon juice
 1 teaspoon Splenda® sweetener
 3 ounces club soda
 Cherry

Shake the vodka, lemon juice and Splenda® sweetener in a shaker with ice and strain into an old-fashioned glass with ice. Add the club soda and stir. Garnish with the cherry.

Nutritional Facts: Protein: 0   Carbohydrates: 2.6 grams
Calories: 138

Vodka Cooler

 2 ounces vodka
 4 ounces diet lemon-lime soda
 Lemon wedge

Mix the vodka and diet lemon-lime soda in an old-fashioned glass with ice and stir. Garnish with the lemon wedge.

Nutritional Facts: Protein: 0   Carbohydrates: 0   Calories: 130

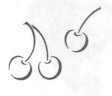

VODKA DRINKS

Vodka Daisy

2 ounces vodka
1 ounce lemon juice
1 teaspoon grenadine (substitute cherry sugar-free syrup)
1/2 teaspoon Splenda® sweetener
Cherry
Orange slice

Shake all the ingredients in a shaker with ice and strain into an old-fashioned glass with ice. Garnish with the cherry and orange slice.

Nutritional Facts: Protein: 0   Carbohydrates: 2.6 grams
Calories: 138

Vodka Sling

2 ounces vodka
2 ounces lemon juice
1 teaspoon Splenda® sweetener
2 teaspoons water
Lemon twist

Shake all the ingredients in a shaker with ice and strain into an old-fashioned glass. Garnish with the lemon twist.

Nutritional Facts: Protein: 0   Carbohydrates: 5.2 grams
Calories: 146

Vodka Sour

  2 ounces vodka
  1 ounce lemon juice
  1/2 teaspoon Splenda® sweetener
  Cherry

Shake all the ingredients in a shaker with ice and strain into an old-fashioned glass with ice. Garnish with the cherry.

Nutritional Facts: Protein: 0   Carbohydrates: 2.6 grams
Calories: 138

Vodka Stinger

  2 ounces vodka
  1/2 ounce crème de menthe sugar-free syrup

Shake all the ingredients in a shaker with ice and strain into a chilled cocktail glass.

Nutritional Facts: Protein: 0   Carbohydrates: 0   Calories: 130

Vodka Swizzle

- 2 ounces vodka
- 1 ounce Rose's Lime Juice
- 2 ounces club soda
- 1 teaspoon Splenda® sweetener
- 2 dashes of bitters

Shake all the ingredients in a shaker with ice and strain into an old-fashioned glass with ice.

Nutritional Facts: Protein: 0   Carbohydrates: 2.8 grams
Calories: 138

Vodka Tonic

- 2 ounces vodka
- Diet tonic
- Lime wedge

Add the vodka and diet tonic to an old-fashioned glass filled with ice and stir. Garnish with the lime wedge.

Nutritional Facts: Protein: 0   Carbohydrates: 0   Calories: 130

White Russian

  2 ounces vodka
  1 ounce light cream
  1 ounce coffee or Kahlua® sugar-free syrup

Shake all the ingredients in a shaker with ice and strain into an old-fashioned glass with ice.

Nutritional Facts: Protein: 1.1 gram   Carbohydrates: 1 gram
Calories: 230

White Wim

  2 ounces vodka
  1 ounce lemon juice
  1 ounce pineapple sugar-free syrup
  Club soda

Shake all the ingredients except the club soda in a shaker with ice and pour into an old-fashioned glass with ice. Top off with the club soda.

Nutritional Facts: Protein: 0   Carbohydrates: 2.6 grams
Calories: 138

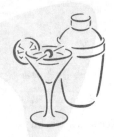

Martini Drinks

Apple Martini

2 ounces vodka
2 ounces sweet 'n' sour mix (sugar-free)
1 ounce green apple sugar-free syrup

Shake all the ingredients in a shaker with ice and strain into a chilled cocktail glass.

Nutritional Facts: Protein: 0   Carbohydrates: 0   Calories: 130

Banana Martini

1 ounce vodka
1 ounce rum
1 ounce banana sugar-free syrup
2 ounces light cream or half & half

Shake all the ingredients in a shaker with ice and strain into a chilled cocktail glass.

Nutritional Facts: Protein: 2 grams   Carbohydrates: 2 grams
Calories: 330

Cajun Martini

  2 ounces vodka
  1 teaspoon dry vermouth
  1 large jalapeño pepper

Shake all the ingredients in a shaker with ice and strain into a chilled cocktail glass. Garnish with the jalapeño pepper.

Nutritional Facts: Protein: 0   Carbohydrates: 0   Calories: 130

Caramel Apple Martini

  2 ounces vodka
  1 ounce green apple sugar-free syrup
  1 ounce caramel sugar-free syrup
  2 ounces light cream or half & half

Shake all the ingredients in a shaker with ice and strain into a chilled cocktail glass.

Nutritional Facts: Protein: 2 grams   Carbohydrates: 2 grams   Calories: 330

Cherry Martini

  2 ounces vodka
  2 ounces sweet 'n' sour mix (sugar-free)
  1 ounce cherry sugar-free syrup

Shake all the ingredients in a shaker with ice and strain into a chilled cocktail glass.

Nutritional Facts: Protein: 0   Carbohydrates: 0   Calories: 130

MARTINI DRINKS

Chocolate Martini

    2 ounces vodka
    2 ounces light cream or half & half
    1 ounce chocolate sugar-free syrup

Shake all the ingredients in a shaker with ice and strain into a chilled cocktail glass.

Nutritional Facts: Protein: 2 grams   Carbohydrates: 2 grams
Calories: 330

Coconut Martini

    2 ounces vodka
    2 ounces light cream or half & half
    1 ounce coconut sugar-free syrup

Shake all the ingredients in a shaker with ice and strain into a chilled cocktail glass.

Nutritional Facts: Protein: 2 grams   Carbohydrates: 2 grams
Calories: 330

Gin or Vodka Martini

2 ounces gin or vodka
1 teaspoon dry vermouth
Cocktail olive
Cocktail onion (optional)

Shake the first two ingredients in a shaker with ice and strain into a chilled cocktail glass. Garnish with the cocktail olive and onion.

Nutritional Facts: Protein: 0   Carbohydrates: 0   Calories: 130

Key Lime Martini

2 ounces vanilla vodka
1 ounce lime sugar-free syrup
2 ounces light cream or half & half

Shake all the ingredients in a shaker with ice and strain into a chilled cocktail glass.

Nutritional Facts: Protein: 2 grams   Carbohydrates: 2 grams
Calories: 130

MARTINI DRINKS

Kiwi Martini

    2 ounces vodka
    2 ounces sweet 'n' sour mix (sugar-free)
    1/4 cup chopped kiwi
    1 ounce kiwi sugar-free syrup
    1 kiwi slice

Combine all the ingredients in a shaker with ice and strain into a chilled cocktail glass. Drop the kiwi slice in the bottom of the glass for garnish.

Nutritional Facts: Protein: 0   Carbohydrates: 0   Calories: 130

Lemon Drop Martini

    2 ounces lemon vodka
    2 ounces sweet 'n' sour mix (sugar-free)
    1 teaspoon Splenda® sweetener

Shake all the ingredients in a shaker with ice and strain into a chilled cocktail glass.

Nutritional Facts: Protein: 0   Carbohydrates: 0   Calories: 130

Mandarin Martini

2 ounces orange vodka

2 ounces sweet 'n' sour mix (sugar-free)

1 teaspoon orange sugar-free syrup

6 segments of mandarin orange

Combine all the ingredients and 4 mandarin orange segments in a shaker with ice. Shake and strain into a chilled cocktail glass. Drop 2 mandarin orange segments in the bottom of the glass for garnish.

Nutritional Facts: Protein: 0   Carbohydrates: 0   Calories: 130

Peach Martini

2 ounces vodka

2 ounces sweet 'n' sour mix (sugar-free)

$1/4$ cup of chopped peaches

1 ounce peach sugar-free syrup

1 peach slice

Combine all the ingredients in a shaker with ice and strain into a chilled cocktail glass. Drop the peach slice in the bottom of the glass for garnish.

Nutritional Facts: Protein: 0   Carbohydrates: 0   Calories: 130

Pineapple Martini

- 2 ounces vodka
- 2 ounces sweet 'n' sour mix (sugar-free)
- 1/4 cup chopped pineapple
- 1 ounce pineapple sugar-free syrup
- 2 pineapple chunks

Combine all the ingredients in a shaker with ice and strain into a chilled cocktail glass. Drop the pineapple chunks in the bottom of the glass for garnish.

Nutritional Facts: Protein: 0   Carbohydrates: 0   Calories: 130

Raspberry Martini

- 2 ounces vodka
- 2 ounces sweet 'n' sour mix (sugar-free)
- 1/4 cup chopped raspberries
- 1 ounce raspberry sugar-free syrup
- 2 raspberries

Combine all the ingredients in a shaker with ice and strain into a chilled cocktail glass. Drop the 2 raspberries in the bottom of the glass for garnish.

Nutritional Facts: Protein: 0   Carbohydrates: 0   Calories: 130

DR. DOUGLAS J. MARKHAM

Root Beer Martini

  2 ounces vanilla vodka
  2 ounces diet root beer
  1 ounce root beer sugar-free syrup

Shake all the ingredients in a shaker with ice and strain into a chilled cocktail glass.

Nutritional Facts: Protein: 0   Carbohydrates: 0   Calories: 130

Strawberry Martini

  2 ounces vodka
  2 ounces sweet 'n' sour mix (sugar-free)
  $\frac{1}{4}$ cup chopped strawberries
  1 ounce strawberry sugar-free syrup
  1 strawberry

Combine all the ingredients in a shaker with ice. Shake and strain into a chilled cocktail glass. Drop the strawberry in the bottom of the glass for garnish.

Nutritional Facts: Protein: 0   Carbohydrates: 0   Calories: 130

Tiramisu Martini

    2 ounces vanilla vodka
    ½ ounce coffee or Kahlua® sugar-free syrup
    ½ ounce Irish cream sugar-free syrup
    1 ounce chocolate sugar-free syrup
    2 ounces light cream or half & half

Shake all the ingredients in a shaker with ice and strain into a chilled cocktail glass.

Nutritional Facts: Protein: 2 grams   Carbohydrates: 2 grams
Calories: 330

Watermelon Martini

    2 ounces vodka
    2 ounces sweet 'n' sour mix (sugar-free)
    ¼ cup chopped watermelon
    1 ounce watermelon sugar-free syrup

Combine all the ingredients in a shaker with ice. Shake and strain into a chilled cocktail glass. Garnish with a small wedge of watermelon.

Nutritional Facts: Protein: 0   Carbohydrates: 0   Calories: 130

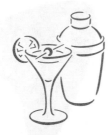

Rum Drinks

Banana Rum

    2 ounces light rum
    $\frac{1}{2}$ ounce banana sugar-free syrup
    $\frac{1}{2}$ ounce orange juice (substitute Sugar-Free Tang® for
        orange juice)

Shake all the ingredients in a shaker with ice and strain into a chilled cocktail glass.

Nutritional Facts: Protein: 0   Carbohydrates: 0   Calories: 130

Banana Rum Cream

    2 ounces dark rum
    1 ounce banana sugar-free syrup
    1 ounce light cream

Shake all the ingredients in a shaker with ice and strain into a chilled cocktail glass.

Nutritional Facts: Protein: 1 gram   Carbohydrates: 1 gram
Calories: 330

Beachcomber

2 ounces light rum
$^1/_2$ ounce Rose's Lime Juice
$^1/_2$ ounce brandy
$^1/_2$ ounce cherry sugar-free syrup
2 teaspoons Splenda® sweetener
Lime wedge

Shake all the ingredients in a shaker with ice and strain into a cocktail glass. Garnish with the lime wedge.

Nutritional Facts: Protein: 0   Carbohydrates: 1.4 grams
Calories: 166

Between the Sheets

1 ounce light rum
1 ounce brandy
$^3/_4$ ounce triple sec (substitute orange sugar-free syrup)
$^1/_2$ ounce lemon juice

Shake all the ingredients in a shaker with ice and strain into a chilled cocktail glass.

Nutritional Facts: Protein: 0   Carbohydrates: 1.3 grams
Calories: 140

Black Devil

  2 ounces light rum
  1/2 ounce dry vermouth

Shake the ingredients in a shaker with ice and strain into a chilled cocktail glass.

Nutritional Facts: Protein: 0   Carbohydrates: 0   Calories: 140

Bolero

  2 ounces anejo rum
  1 ounce sweet vermouth
  1 ounce green apple sugar-free syrup
  Dash of bitters

Shake all the ingredients in a shaker with ice and strain into an old-fashioned glass over crushed ice.

Nutritional Facts: Protein: 0   Carbohydrates: 0   Calories: 150

Boston Sidecar

  1 ounce light rum
  1 ounce brandy
  1/2 ounce triple sec (substitute orange sugar-free syrup)
  1/2 ounce lemon juice

Shake all the ingredients in a shaker with ice and strain into a chilled cocktail glass.

Nutritional Facts: Protein: 0   Carbohydrates: 1.3 grams
Calories: 140

Brown Cocktail

1 ounce dark rum
$^1/_2$ ounce dry vermouth
1 ounce gin

Shake all the ingredients in a shaker with ice and strain into a chilled cocktail glass.

Nutritional Facts: Protein: 0   Carbohydrates: 0   Calories: 140

Buccaneer Cocktail

$1^1/_2$ ounces light rum
$1^1/_2$ ounces dark rum
1 ounce coffee or Kahlua® sugar-free syrup
1 ounce pineapple sugar-free syrup
1 ounce heavy cream
Nutmeg

Combine the first 4 ingredients in a shaker with ice and strain into a wineglass with crushed ice. Top with the heavy cream and sprinkle with the nutmeg.

Nutritional Facts: Protein: 1 gram   Carbohydrates: 1 gram
Calories: 295

Cardinal

2 ounces light rum
1/2 ounce amaretto sugar-free syrup
1/2 ounce triple sec (substitute orange sugar-free syrup)
1/2 ounce Rose's Lime Juice
1/2 teaspoon grenadine (substitute cherry sugar-free syrup)
Lime slice

Shake all the ingredients in a shaker with ice and strain into a chilled cocktail glass. Garnish with the lime slice.

Nutritional Facts: Protein: 0   Carbohydrates: 1.4 grams
Calories: 134

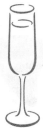

Chocolate Rum

1 ounce dark rum
1/2 ounce 151 proof rum
1/2 ounce chocolate sugar-free syrup
1/2 ounce crème de menthe sugar-free syrup
1/2 ounce light cream

Shake all the ingredients in a shaker with ice and strain into a chilled cocktail glass.

Nutritional Facts: Protein: 0.5 grams   Carbohydrates: 0.5 grams
Calories: 142.5

RUM DRINKS

Continental

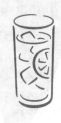

  2 ounces light rum
  ¹/₂ ounce Rose's Lime Juice
  ¹/₂ ounce lemon juice
  1 ounce crème de menthe sugar-free syrup
  ¹/₂ ounce simple syrup (sugar-free)
  Lemon twist

Shake all the ingredients in a shaker with ice and strain into a chilled cocktail glass. Garnish with the lemon twist.

Nutritional Facts: Protein: 0   Carbohydrates: 2.7 grams
Calories: 138

Cosmos

  2 ounces light rum
  1 ounce Rose's Lime Juice
  1 teaspoon Splenda® sweetener
  Lemon twist

Shake all the ingredients in a shaker with ice and strain into a chilled cocktail glass. Garnish with the lemon twist.

Nutritional Facts: Protein: 0   Carbohydrates: 2.8 grams
Calories: 138

Creole

2 ounces light rum
3 ounces beef bouillon
$\frac{1}{2}$ ounce lemon juice
Salt
Pepper
Dash of Tabasco sauce
Lemon twist

Shake all the ingredients in a shaker with ice and strain into a chilled cocktail glass. Garnish with the lemon twist.

Nutritional Facts: Protein: 1 gram   Carbohydrates: 2.6 grams
Calories: 138

Cuba Libre

$1\frac{1}{2}$ ounces light rum
Diet cola
$\frac{1}{4}$ lime

Mix the rum and diet cola in an old-fashioned glass with ice. Squeeze the lime on top and stir.

Nutritional Facts: Protein: 0   Carbohydrates: 1.4 grams
Calories: 97.5

Cuban Cocktail

>2 ounces light rum
>$^1/_2$ ounce Rose's Lime Juice
>$^1/_2$ ounce lemon juice
>$^1/_2$ teaspoon Splenda® sweetener
>Lemon twist

Shake all the ingredients in a shaker with ice and strain into a chilled cocktail glass. Garnish with the lemon twist.

Nutritional Facts: Protein: 0   Carbohydrates: 2.7 grams
Calories: 138

Davis Cocktail

>1$^1/_2$ ounces dark rum
>$^3/_4$ ounce dry vermouth
>$^1/_2$ ounce raspberry sugar-free syrup
>Juice of $^1/_2$ lime

Shake all the ingredients in a shaker with ice and strain into a chilled cocktail glass.

Nutritional Facts: Protein: 0   Carbohydrates: 1.4 grams
Calories: 110

Derby Special

- 2 ounces light rum
- 1/2 ounce triple sec (substitute orange sugar-free syrup)
- 1 ounce orange juice (substitute Sugar-Free Tang® for orange juice)
- 1/2 ounce Rose's Lime Juice

Blend all the ingredients in a blender with ice and pour into a chilled cocktail glass.

Nutritional Facts: Protein: 0   Carbohydrates: 1.4 grams
Calories: 134

Ernest Hemingway Special

- 2 ounces light rum
- Juice of 1/2 lime
- 1/2 ounce grapefruit juice (substitute Crystal Light® Ruby Red Grapefruit for grapefruit juice)
- 1/2 ounce cherry sugar-free syrup

Shake all the ingredients in a shaker with ice and strain into a chilled cocktail glass.

Nutritional Facts: Protein: 0   Carbohydrates: 1.4 grams
Calories: 134

Fireman's Sour

2 ounces light rum
1 ounce Rose's Lime Juice
$\frac{1}{2}$ ounce grenadine (substitute cherry sugar-free syrup)
1 ounce club soda
Cherry
Lemon slice

Shake the rum, Rose's Lime Juice and cherry sugar-free syrup in shaker with ice and strain into an old-fashioned glass with crushed ice. Add the club soda and stir. Garnish with the cherry and lemon slice.

Nutritional Facts: Protein: 0   Carbohydrates: 2.8 grams
Calories: 138

Havana Cocktail

2 ounces light rum
1 ounce pineapple sugar-free syrup
$\frac{1}{2}$ ounce lemon juice

Shake all the ingredients in a shaker with ice and strain into a chilled cocktail glass.

Nutritional Facts: Protein: 0   Carbohydrates: 1.3 grams
Calories: 134

Immaculate

2 ounces light rum
$^1/_2$ ounce amaretto sugar-free syrup
$^1/_2$ ounce Rose's Lime Juice
$^1/_2$ ounce lemon juice
$^1/_2$ teaspoon Splenda® sweetener

Shake all the ingredients in a shaker with ice and strain into a chilled cocktail glass.

Nutritional Facts: Protein: 0   Carbohydrates: 2.7 grams
Calories: 138

Jamaican Fizz

2 ounces dark rum
1 ounce pineapple sugar-free syrup
1 teaspoon Splenda® sweetener
4 ounces club soda

Shake the rum, pineapple sugar-free syrup and Splenda® sweetener in a shaker with ice and strain into an old-fashioned glass with crushed ice. Add the club soda and stir.

Nutritional Facts: Protein: 0   Carbohydrates: 0   Calories: 130

Mary Pickford

2 ounces light rum
1 ounce pineapple sugar-free syrup
$^1/_2$ teaspoon cherry sugar-free syrup
Cherry

Shake all the ingredients in a shaker with ice and strain into a chilled cocktail glass. Garnish with the cherry.

Nutritional Facts: Protein: 0   Carbohydrates: 0   Calories: 130

Mojito

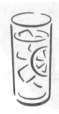

1 teaspoon Splenda® sweetener
Juice of $^1/_2$ lime
3 whole mint leaves
2 ounces light rum
Club soda
Sprig of mint

Place the Splenda® sweetener and lime juice in an old-fashioned glass and stir until dissolved. Add the mint leaves and crush them in the glass. Fill the glass with crushed ice and the rum while stirring gently. Top off with the club soda and garnish with a sprig of mint.

Nutritional Facts: Protein: 0   Carbohydrates: 1.4 grams
Calories: 134

Monkey Wrench

    2 ounces light rum
    3 ounces grapefruit juice (substitute Crystal Light® Ruby Red
        Grapefruit for grapefruit juice)
    Dash of bitters

Shake all the ingredients in a shaker with ice and strain into an old-fashioned glass with crushed ice.

Nutritional Facts: Protein: 0   Carbohydrates: 0   Calories: 130

Nevada Cocktail

    2 ounces light rum
    2 ounces grapefruit juice (substitute Crystal Light® Ruby Red
        Grapefruit for grapefruit juice)
    1 ounce Rose's Lime Juice
    2 teaspoons Splenda® sweetener
    Dash of bitters

Shake all the ingredients in a shaker with ice and strain into a chilled cocktail glass.

Nutritional Facts: Protein: 0   Carbohydrates: 2.8 grams
Calories: 138

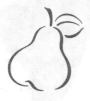

Pineapple Cocktail

2 ounces light rum
1 ounce pineapple sugar-free syrup
$1/2$ ounce lemon juice

Shake all the ingredients in a shaker with ice and strain into a chilled cocktail glass.

Nutritional Facts: Protein: 0   Carbohydrates: 1.3 grams
Calories: 134

Pineapple Fizz

2 ounces light rum
1 ounce pineapple sugar-free syrup
$1/2$ teaspoon Splenda® sweetener
Club soda

Shake the rum, sugar-free pineapple syrup and Splenda® sweetener in a shaker with ice and strain into an old-fashioned glass with crushed ice. Fill the glass with club soda.

Nutritional Facts: Protein: 0   Carbohydrates: 0   Calories: 130

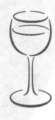

Planter's Punch

   1½ ounces dark rum
   1½ ounces light rum
   3 ounces orange juice (substitute Sugar-Free Tang® for
      orange juice)
   ½ ounce Rose's Lime Juice
   Simple syrup (sugar-free) to taste
   Orange slice
   Pineapple chunk
   Maraschino cherry

Shake all the ingredients in a shaker with ice and strain into an old-fashioned glass with ice. Garnish with the fruit speared with a toothpick. Serve with a straw.

Nutritional Facts: Protein: 0   Carbohydrates: 1.4 grams
Calories: 199

Rum Fizz

   2 ounces light rum
   1 ounce lemon juice
   1 teaspoon Splenda® sweetener
   4 ounces club soda

Shake the rum, lemon juice and Splenda® sweetener in a shaker with ice and strain into an old-fashioned glass with crushed ice. Fill the glass with club soda and stir.

Nutritional Facts: Protein: 0   Carbohydrates: 2.6 grams
Calories: 138

Rum Martini

    2 ounces light rum
    1/2 ounce dry vermouth
    Cocktail olive

Shake all the ingredients in a shaker and strain into a chilled cocktail glass. Garnish with the cocktail olive.

Nutritional Facts: Protein: 0   Carbohydrates: 0   Calories: 140

Rum Cocktail

    2 ounces light rum
    1 ounce Rose's Lime Juice
    1 teaspoon grenadine (substitute cherry sugar-free syrup)

Shake all the ingredients in a shaker with ice and strain into a chilled cocktail glass.

Nutritional Facts: Protein: 0   Carbohydrates: 2.8 grams
Calories: 138

Rum Milk Punch

    2 ounces light rum
    2 ounces light cream or half & half
    1 teaspoon Splenda® sweetener
    ¼ teaspoon nutmeg

Shake all the ingredients in a shaker with ice and strain into an old-fashioned glass with ice. Garnish with the nutmeg.

Nutritional Facts: Protein: 2 grams   Carbohydrates: 2 grams
Calories: 230

Rum Screwdriver

    2 ounces light rum
    5 ounces orange juice (substitute Sugar-Free Tang® for
        orange juice)

Shake all the ingredients in a shaker with ice and strain into an old-fashioned glass with crushed ice.

Nutritional Facts: Protein: 0   Carbohydrates: 0   Calories: 130

Rum Sour

>   2 ounces light rum
>   1 ounce lemon juice
>   ½ ounce simple syrup (sugar-free)
>   Cherry
>   Orange slice

Shake all the ingredients in a shaker with ice and strain into a chilled cocktail glass. Garnish with the cherry and orange slice.

Nutritional Facts: Protein: 0   Carbohydrates: 2.6 grams
Calories: 138

Rum Swizzle

>   2 ounces light rum
>   ½ ounce Rose's Lime Juice
>   1 teaspoon Splenda® sweetener
>   Dash of bitters
>   3 ounces club soda

Shake the rum, Rose's Lime Juice, Splenda® sweetener and bitters in a shaker with ice and strain into an old-fashioned glass with crushed ice. Add the club soda and stir. Serve with a swizzle stick.

Nutritional Facts: Protein: 0   Carbohydrates: 1.4 grams
Calories: 134

Saxon Cocktail

2 ounces light rum
1 ounce lime juice
1 teaspoon grenadine (substitute cherry sugar-free syrup)
Orange slice

Shake all the ingredients in a shaker with ice and strain into a chilled cocktail glass. Garnish with the orange slice.

Nutritional Facts: Protein: 0   Carbohydrates: 2.8 grams
Calories: 138

Scorpion

2 ounces anejo rum
1 ounce brandy
1 ounce lemon juice
2 ounces orange juice (substitute Sugar-Free Tang® for orange juice)
$^1/_2$ ounce orgeat (substitute almond sugar-free syrup)
Cherry
Orange slice

Blend all the ingredients in a blender with ice until smooth and pour into an old-fashioned glass. Garnish with the cherry and orange slice. Serve with a straw.

Nutritional Facts: Protein: 0   Carbohydrates: 2.6 grams
Calories: 142

Serpentine

2 ounces light rum
1 ounce brandy
1 ounce sweet vermouth
1 ounce lemon juice
$\frac{1}{2}$ teaspoon Splenda® sweetener

Shake all the ingredients in a shaker with ice and strain into a chilled cocktail glass.

Nutritional Facts: Protein: 0   Carbohydrates: 2.6 grams
Calories: 229

Spiced Rum or Rum and Diet Cola

2 ounces spiced rum or light rum
6 ounces diet cola
Lime slice

Pour all the ingredients into an old-fashioned glass with crushed ice. Garnish with the lime slice.

Nutritional Facts: Protein: 0   Carbohydrates: 0   Calories: 130

Tahiti Club

- 2 ounces light rum
- $1/2$ ounce lemon juice
- $1/2$ ounce lime juice
- $1/2$ ounce pineapple sugar-free syrup
- $1/2$ ounce cherry sugar-free syrup
- Lemon slice

Shake all the ingredients in a shaker with ice and strain into an old-fashioned glass with crushed ice. Garnish with the lemon slice.

Nutritional Facts: Protein: 0   Carbohydrates: 2.7 grams
Calories: 138

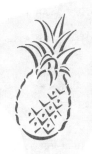

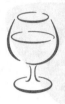

Scotch Whisky Drinks

Affinity

    2 ounces Scotch
    1$^1/_2$ ounces sweet vermouth
    1$^1/_2$ ounces dry vermouth
    Several dashes orange bitters

Shake all the ingredients in a shaker with ice and strain into a chilled cocktail glass.

Nutritional Facts: Protein: 0   Carbohydrates: 2 grams
Calories: 188

Black Jack

    2 ounces Scotch
    1 ounce lemon juice
    1 coffee or Kahlua® sugar-free syrup
    1 ounce triple sec (substitute orange sugar-free syrup)

Shake all the ingredients in a shaker with ice and strain into a chilled cocktail glass.

Nutritional Facts: Protein: 0   Carbohydrates: 2.6 grams
Calories: 136

Blimey

    2 ounces Scotch

    1 ounce Rose's Lime Juice

    ½ teaspoon Splenda® sweetener

Shake all the ingredients in a shaker with ice and strain into a chilled cocktail glass.

Nutritional Facts: Protein: 0   Carbohydrates: 2.8 grams
Calories: 138

Blinder

    2 ounces Scotch

    5 ounces grapefruit juice (substitute Crystal Light® Ruby Red
       Grapefruit for grapefruit juice)

    1 teaspoon grenadine (substitute cherry sugar-free syrup)

Shake all the ingredients in a shaker with ice and strain into a chilled cocktail glass. Add the teaspoon of grenadine to the top.

Nutritional Facts: Protein: 0   Carbohydrates: 0   Calories: 128

Fancy Scotch

    2 ounces Scotch
    $1/2$ ounce triple sec (substitute orange sugar-free syrup)
    $1/2$ teaspoon Splenda® sweetener
    Several dashes of bitters
    Lemon twist

Shake all the ingredients in a shaker with ice and strain into a chilled cocktail glass. Garnish with the lemon twist.

Nutritional Facts: Protein: 0   Carbohydrates: 0   Calories: 128

Godfather

    2 ounces Scotch
    1 ounce amaretto sugar-free syrup

Shake all the ingredients in a shaker with ice and strain into an old-fashioned glass with crushed ice.

Nutritional Facts: Protein: 0   Carbohydrates: 0   Calories: 128

Harry Lauder

    $1^1/2$ ounces Scotch
    $1^1/2$ ounces sweet vermouth
    $1/2$ teaspoon Splenda® sweetener

Shake all the ingredients in a shaker with ice and strain into a chilled cocktail glass.

Nutritional Facts: Protein: 0   Carbohydrates: 1 gram
Calories: 126

Hawaiian Bull

 1½ ounces Scotch
 ½ ounce orgeat (substitute almond sugar-free syrup)
 Pineapple chunk

Pour the Scotch into an old-fashioned glass filled with crushed ice and top off with the orgeat. Garnish with the pineapple chunk.

Nutritional Facts: Protein: 0   Carbohydrates: 0   Calories: 96

Highland

 2 ounces Scotch
 3 ounces light cream or half & half
 1 teaspoon Splenda® sweetener
 Nutmeg

Shake all the ingredients in a shaker with ice and strain into an old-fashioned glass with crushed ice. Sprinkle the nutmeg on top.

Nutritional Facts: Protein: 3 grams   Carbohydrates: 3 grams
Calories: 428

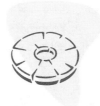

Highland Fling

2 ounces Scotch
1 ounce lemon juice
1 ounce water
1 teaspoon Splenda® sweetener
Lemon twist

Shake all the ingredients in a shaker with ice and strain into a chilled cocktail glass. Garnish with the lemon twist.

Nutritional Facts: Protein: 0   Carbohydrates: 2.6 grams
Calories: 136

Horseshoe

1 lemon peel (peeled in long spiral)
3 ounces Scotch
½ ounce sweet vermouth
½ ounce dry vermouth

Place the lemon peel in an old-fashioned glass, leaving one end of the peel hanging over the rim. Fill the glass with crushed ice. Shake all the ingredients in a shaker with ice and strain into the glass.

Nutritional Facts: Protein: 0   Carbohydrates: 0   Calories: 212

Jock Collins

  2 ounces Scotch
  3 ounces club soda
  1 ounce lemon juice
  1 teaspoon Splenda® sweetener
  Cherry

Shake all the ingredients in a shaker with ice and strain into an old-fashioned glass with crushed ice. Garnish with the cherry.

Nutritional Facts: Protein: 0   Carbohydrates: 2.6 grams
Calories: 136

McDuff

  2 ounces Scotch
  1 ounce triple sec (substitute orange sugar-free syrup)
  Several dashes of bitters
  Orange slice

Shake all the ingredients in a shaker with ice and strain into a chilled cocktail glass. Garnish with the orange slice.

Nutritional Facts: Protein: 0   Carbohydrates: 0   Calories: 128

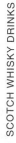

SCOTCH WHISKY DRINKS

Miami Beach

> 1 ounce Scotch
>
> 1 ounce dry vermouth
>
> 1 ounce grapefruit juice (substitute Crystal Light® Ruby Red Grapefruit for grapefruit juice)

Shake all the ingredients in a shaker with ice and strain into a chilled cocktail glass.

Nutritional Facts: Protein: 0   Carbohydrates: 0   Calories: 74

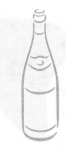

Rob Roy

> 2 ounces Scotch
>
> 1 teaspoon sweet vermouth
>
> Cherry

Shake all the ingredients in a shaker with ice and strain into a chilled cocktail glass. Garnish with the cherry.

Nutritional Facts: Protein: 0   Carbohydrates: 0   Calories: 128

Saucy Sue

> 2 ounces Scotch
> ¼ ounce Rose's Lime Juice
> 3 ounces diet ginger ale
> Lemon wedge

Shake all the ingredients in a shaker with ice and strain into an old-fashioned glass with crushed ice. Garnish with the lemon wedge.

Nutritional Facts: Protein: 0   Carbohydrates: 0.6 grams
Calories: 130

Scotch Cobbler

> 2 ounces Scotch
> 3 ounces club soda
> 1 teaspoon Splenda® sweetener
> Cherry
> Orange slice

Shake all the ingredients in a shaker with ice and strain into an old-fashioned glass with crushed ice. Garnish with the cherry and orange slice.

Nutritional Facts: Protein: 0   Carbohydrates: 0   Calories: 128

Scotch Cooler

2 ounces Scotch
4 ounces diet lemon-lime soda
Lemon wedge

Shake all the ingredients in a shaker with ice and strain into an old-fashioned glass with crushed ice. Garnish with the lemon wedge.

Nutritional Facts: Protein: 0   Carbohydrates: 0   Calories: 128

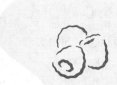

Scotch Old-Fashioned

2 ounces Scotch
$1/4$ ounce 151 proof rum
$1/2$ teaspoon Splenda® sweetener
Dash of bitters
Lime wedge

Shake all the ingredients in a shaker with ice and strain into an old-fashioned glass with crushed ice. Garnish with the lime wedge.

Nutritional Facts: Protein: 0   Carbohydrates: 0   Calories: 160.5

Scotch Nectar

    2 ounces Scotch
    1/2 ounce peach sugar-free syrup
    1/4 ounce fresh lemon juice
    1/2 ounce green apple sugar-free syrup
    Peach slice

Shake all the ingredients in a shaker with ice and strain into a chilled cocktail glass. Garnish with the peach slice.

Nutritional Facts: Protein: 0   Carbohydrates: 0.6 grams
Calories: 130

Scotch Sour

    2 ounces Scotch
    1 ounce lemon juice
    1 teaspoon simple syrup (sugar-free)
    Cherry
    Orange slice

Shake all the ingredients in a shaker with ice and strain into a chilled cocktail glass. Garnish with the cherry and orange slice.

Nutritional Facts: Protein: 0   Carbohydrates: 2.6 grams
Calories: 136

Tartan Swizzle

1¹/₂ ounces Scotch
¹/₂ ounce Rose's Lime Juice
1 teaspoon Splenda® sweetener
Several dashes of bitters
3 ounces club soda

Shake all the ingredients except the club soda in a shaker with ice and strain into an old-fashioned glass with crushed ice. Top off with the club soda and stir.

Nutritional Facts: Protein: 0   Carbohydrates: 1.4 grams
Calories: 96

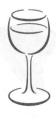

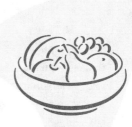

Tequila Drinks

Be Merry

    1¹/₂ ounces tequila

    1 tablespoon raspberry sugar-free syrup

    2 teaspoons lemon juice

    Dash of triple sec (substitute orange sugar-free syrup)

    Orange slice

Shake all the ingredients in a shaker with ice and strain into a chilled cocktail glass. Garnish with the orange slice.

Nutritional Facts: Protein: 0   Carbohydrates: 1.3 grams
Calories: 97.5

Bravo Bull

    2 ounces tequila

    1 ounce coffee or Kahlua® sugar-free syrup

Shake all the ingredients in a shaker with ice and strain into an old-fashioned glass with ice.

Nutritional Facts: Protein: 0   Carbohydrates: 0   Calories: 130

Bunny

 2 ounces tequila
 1 ounce green apple sugar-free syrup
 ½ ounce lemon juice
 1 teaspoon maple sugar-free syrup
 Several dashes of triple sec (substitute orange sugar-free syrup)
 Lemon slice

Shake all the ingredients in a shaker with ice and strain into an old-fashioned glass with ice. Garnish with the lemon slice.

Nutritional Facts: Protein: 0   Carbohydrates: 1.3 grams Calories: 134

California Dream

 2 ounces tequila
 1 ounce dry vermouth
 1 ounce sweet vermouth
 Cherry

Shake all the ingredients in a shaker with ice and strain into a chilled cocktail glass. Garnish with the cherry.

Nutritional Facts: Protein: 0   Carbohydrates: 1 gram Calories: 170

Changuirongo

  2 ounces tequila
  4 ounces diet ginger ale
  Lime wedge

Pour the tequila and diet ginger ale into an old-fashioned glass with ice and stir. Garnish with the lime wedge.

Nutritional Facts: Protein: 0   Carbohydrates: 0   Calories: 130

Coco Loco

  1 coconut
  1 ounce tequila
  1 ounce gin
  1 ounce light rum
  1 ounce pineapple sugar-free syrup
  ½ fresh lime

Saw off the top of the coconut. Leave the coconut water in the husk, add ice and all the ingredients. Squeeze the lime over the drink, drop it in and stir.

Nutritional Facts: Protein: 0   Carbohydrates: 1.4 grams
Calories: 199

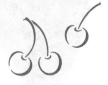

Cosmorita

2 ounces tequila

3/4 ounce triple sec (substitute orange sugar-free syrup)

2 ounces cranberry juice (Ocean Spray® Light Cranberry Juice Cocktail)

3/4 ounce fresh lime juice

Lime wedge

Shake all the ingredients in a shaker with ice and strain into a chilled cocktail glass. Garnish with the lime wedge.

Nutritional Facts: Protein: 0   Carbohydrates: 6 grams
Calories: 150

Doralto

2 ounces tequila

1 ounce lemon juice

1 teaspoon Splenda® sweetener

Dash of bitters

4 ounces diet tonic water

Lime wedge

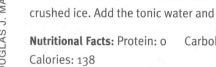

Shake the tequila, lemon juice, Splenda® sweetener, and bitters in a shaker with ice and strain into an old-fashioned glass over crushed ice. Add the tonic water and garnish with the lime wedge.

Nutritional Facts: Protein: 0   Carbohydrates: 2.6 grams
Calories: 138

El Cid

  2 ounces tequila
  1 ounce Rose's Lime Juice
  1 ounce orgeat (substitute almond sugar-free syrup)
  Grenadine (substitute cherry sugar-free syrup)
  Tonic water
  Lime slice

Pour the tequila, lime juice and almond sugar-free syrup into an old-fashioned glass and stir. Add crushed ice and top off with the tonic water and several dashes of cherry sugar-free syrup. Garnish with the lime slice.

Nutritional Facts: Protein: 0   Carbohydrates: 2.8 grams
Calories: 138

Gentle Ben

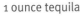

  1 ounce tequila
  1 ounce vodka
  1 ounce gin
  3 ounces orange juice (substitute Sugar-Free Tang® for
      orange juice)
  Orange slice

Shake all the ingredients in a shaker with ice and strain into an old-fashioned glass with ice. Garnish with the orange slice.

Nutritional Facts: Protein: 0   Carbohydrates: 0   Calories: 195

Gentle Bull

2 ounces tequila
1 ounce coffee or Kahlua® sugar-free syrup
1 ounce heavy cream

Shake all the ingredients in a shaker with ice and strain into an old-fashioned glass with crushed ice.

Nutritional Facts: Protein: 1 gram   Carbohydrates: 1 gram
Calories: 230

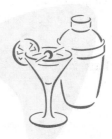

Horny Bull

2 ounces tequila
4 ounces orange juice (substitute Sugar-Free Tang® for orange juice)

Shake all the ingredients in a shaker with ice and strain into an old-fashioned glass filled with ice.

Nutritional Facts: Protein: 0   Carbohydrates: 0   Calories: 130

Margarita

Lime slice
Coarse salt
2 ounces tequila
½ ounce triple sec (substitute orange
   sugar-free syrup)
2 ounces sweet 'n' sour mix (sugar-free)
Dash of Rose's Lime Juice

Moisten the rim of a cocktail glass with the lime slice and press the rim into the salt. Shake all the ingredients in a shaker with ice and strain into a chilled cocktail glass.

Nutritional Facts: Protein: 0   Carbohydrates: 0   Calories: 130

Matador

Coarse salt
1½ ounces tequila
½ ounce triple sec or sugar-free orange syrup
Juice of 1 small lime

Moisten the rim of a cocktail glass and press the rim into the coarse salt. Shake all the ingredients in a shaker and strain into the salted cocktail glass.

Nutritional Facts: Protein: 0   Carbohydrates: 2.8 grams
Calories: 101.5

TEQUILA DRINKS

Rocky Point

1½ ounces tequila

3 ounces grapefruit juice (substitute Crystal Light® Ruby Red
  Grapefruit for grapefruit juice)

1 teaspoon orgeat (substitute almond sugar-free syrup)

Dash of Rose's Lime Juice

Dash of triple sec (substitute orange sugar-free syrup)

Mint sprigs

Shake all the ingredients in a shaker with ice and strain into a chilled wineglass. Garnish with the mint sprigs.

Nutritional Facts: Protein: 0   Carbohydrates: 0   Calories: 97.5

Shady Lady

2 ounces tequila

1 ounce watermelon sugar-free syrup

5 ounces grapefruit juice (substitute Crystal Light® Ruby Red
  Grapefruit for grapefruit juice)

Shake all the ingredients in a shaker with ice and strain into an old-fashioned glass with crushed ice.

Nutritional Facts: Protein: 0   Carbohydrates: 0   Calories: 130

Shaker

- 2 ounces tequila
- 1 ounce lemon juice
- 2 ounces pineapple sugar-free syrup
- 1 teaspoon grenadine (substitute cherry sugar-free syrup)

Shake all the ingredients in a shaker with ice and strain into a chilled cocktail glass.

Nutritional Facts: Protein: 0   Carbohydrates: 2.6 grams
Calories: 138

Sno-Cap

- 2 ounces tequila
- 3 ounces cream of coconut (sugar-free)
- 2 tablespoons Rose's Lime Juice
- Lime wedge

Blend all the ingredients in a blender with ice until smooth. Pour into a chilled cocktail glass and garnish with the lime wedge.

Nutritional Facts: Protein: 0   Carbohydrates: 2.8 grams
Calories: 238

Speedy Gonzalez

1½ ounces tequila

3 ounces grapefruit juice (substitute Crystal Light® Ruby Red
Grapefruit for grapefruit juice)

1 teaspoon Splenda® sweetener

Club soda

Shake all the ingredients except the club soda in a shaker with ice and strain into an old-fashioned glass with crushed ice. Top off with club soda.

Nutritional Facts: Protein: 0   Carbohydrates: 0   Calories: 97.5

Tequila Collins

2 ounces tequila

1 ounce lemon juice

1 teaspoon Splenda® sweetener

4 ounces club soda

Cherry

Orange slice

Shake the tequila, lemon juice and Splenda® sweetener in a shaker with ice and strain into an old-fashioned glass with crushed ice. Add the club soda and garnish with the cherry and orange slice. Serve with a straw.

Nutritional Facts: Protein: 0   Carbohydrates: 2.6 grams
Calories: 65

Tequila Julep

    4 mint sprigs
    1 teaspoon Splenda® sweetener
    2 ounces tequila
    4 ounces club soda

Crush 3 mint sprigs in an old-fashioned glass with the Splenda® sweetener. Add the tequila and stir. Add crushed ice and top off with the club soda. Garnish with the mint sprig.

Nutritional Facts: Protein: 0   Carbohydrates: 0   Calories: 130

Tequila Manhattan

    1½ ounces tequila
    ¾ ounce sweet vermouth
    Several splashes of bitters
    1 maraschino cherry

Shake all the ingredients in a shaker with ice and strain into a chilled cocktail glass. Garnish with the cherry.

Nutritional Facts: Protein: 0   Carbohydrates: 0   Calories: 112.5

TEQUILA DRINKS

Tequila Martini

2 ounces tequila
½ ounce dry vermouth
Cocktail olive

Shake all the ingredients in a shaker with ice and strain into a chilled cocktail glass. Garnish with the cocktail olive.

Nutritional Facts: Protein: 0   Carbohydrates: 0   Calories: 140

Tequila Mockingbird

2 ounces tequila
½ ounce lemon juice
1 teaspoon crème de menthe sugar-free syrup

Shake all the ingredients in a shaker with ice and strain into a chilled cocktail glass.

Nutritional Facts: Protein: 0   Carbohydrates: 1.3 grams
Calories: 134

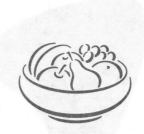

Tequila Sour

    2 ounces tequila
    1 ounce lemon juice
    $\frac{1}{2}$ teaspoon Splenda® sweetener
    Cherry
    Orange slice

Shake all the ingredients in a shaker with ice and strain into a chilled cocktail glass. Garnish with the cherry and orange slice.

Nutritional Facts: Protein: 0   Carbohydrates: 2.6 grams Calories: 138

Tequila Stinger

    2 ounces tequila
    1 ounce crème de menthe sugar-free syrup

Shake all the ingredients in a shaker with ice and strain into a chilled cocktail glass.

Nutritional Facts: Protein: 0   Carbohydrates: 0   Calories: 130

Tequila Sunrise

    2 ounces tequila
    3 ounces orange juice (substitute Sugar-Free Tang® for
        orange juice)
    1 ounce grenadine (substitute cherry sugar-free syrup)

Shake all the ingredients in a shaker with ice and strain into an old-fashioned glass with crushed ice.

Nutritional Facts: Protein: 0   Carbohydrates: 0   Calories: 130

TNT (Tequila 'n' Tonic)

> 2 ounces tequila
> 4 ounces diet tonic
> Lime wedge

Pour the tequila and diet tonic in an old-fashioned glass with ice and stir. Garnish with the lime wedge.

Nutritional Facts: Protein: 0   Carbohydrates: 0   Calories: 130

Viva Villa

> 2 ounces tequila
> ½ ounce Rose's Lime Juice
> ½ ounce lemon juice
> 1 teaspoon Splenda® sweetener
> Lime wedge

Shake all the ingredients in a shaker with ice and strain into a chilled cocktail glass. Garnish with the lime wedge.

Nutritional Facts: Protein: 0   Carbohydrates: 2.7 grams
Calories: 138

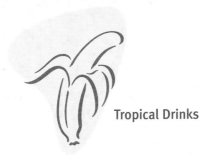

Tropical Drinks

Banana Colada

    1 ounce dark rum
    1 ounce light rum
    1 ounce pineapple sugar-free syrup
    2 ounces cream of coconut (sugar-free)
    1 ounce banana sugar-free syrup
    Cherry

Combine all the ingredients in a blender with ice and blend until smooth. Pour into a wineglass and garnish with the cherry.

Nutritional Facts: Protein: 0   Carbohydrates: 0   Calories: 230

Banana Daiquiri

    2 ounces light rum
    ½ ounce triple sec (substitute orange sugar-free syrup)
    ½ teaspoon Splenda® sweetener
    1 ounce banana sugar-free syrup

Combine all the ingredients in a blender with ice and blend until smooth. Pour into a wineglass.

Nutritional Facts: Protein: 0   Carbohydrates: 0   Calories: 130

Banana Foster

>2 ounces dark rum
>1 ounce banana sugar-free syrup
>1/2 ounce vanilla sugar-free syrup
>2 ounces heavy cream

Combine all the ingredients in a blender with ice and blend until smooth. Pour into a wineglass.

Nutritional Facts: Protein: 2 grams   Carbohydrates: 2 grams
Calories: 465

Banana Smoothie

>1 1/2 ounces light rum
>1 ounce banana sugar-free syrup
>1/2 ounce Rose's Lime Juice
>1/2 ounce yogurt
>1 teaspoon Splenda® sweetener

Combine all the ingredients in a blender with ice and blend until smooth. Pour into a wineglass.

Nutritional Facts: Protein: 1 gram   Carbohydrates: 1 gram
Calories: 100

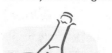

Frozen Daiquiri

    2 ounces light rum
    1 ounce Rose's Lime Juice
    1 ounce triple sec (substitute orange sugar-free syrup)
    1 teaspoon Splenda® sweetener
    Cherry

Combine all the ingredients in a blender with ice and blend until smooth. Pour into a wineglass and garnish with the cherry.

Nutritional Facts: Protein: 0   Carbohydrates: 2.8 grams
Calories: 138

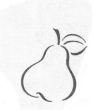

Frozen Fruit Daiquiri

    1½ ounces light rum
    ½ ounce sweet 'n' sour mix (sugar-free)
    ½ ounce heavy cream
    1 ounce appropriate fruit-flavored sugar-free syrup (peach, strawberry, pineapple)
    ¼ cup favorite fruit (peaches, strawberries, pineapple)

Combine all the ingredients in a blender with ice and blend until smooth. Pour into a wineglass.

Nutritional Facts: Protein: 1 gram   Carbohydrates: 5.5 grams
Calories: 187.5

Frozen Margarita

2 ounces tequila
2 ounces sweet 'n' sour mix (sugar-free)
1/2 ounce triple sec (substitute orange sugar-free syrup)
Dash of Rose's Lime Juice
Lime slice

Combine all the ingredients in a blender with ice and blend until smooth. Pour into a chilled cocktail glass and garnish with the lime slice.

Nutritional Facts: Protein: 0   Carbohydrates: 0   Calories: 130

Frozen Fruit Margarita

1 1/2 ounces tequila
1/2 ounce sweet 'n' sour mix (sugar-free)
1 ounce appropriate fruit-flavored sugar-free syrup (peach, strawberry, pineapple)
1/4 cup appropriate fruit (peaches, strawberries, pineapple)
Dash of Rose's Lime Juice

Combine all the ingredients in a blender with ice and blend until smooth. Pour into a chilled cocktail glass.

Nutritional Facts: Protein: 0   Carbohydrates: 4.5 grams Calories: 137.5

Frozen Matador

    2 ounces tequila
    1 ounce pineapple sugar-free syrup
    2 teaspoons Rose's Lime Juice

Combine all the ingredients in a blender with ice and blend until smooth. Pour into a wineglass.

Nutritional Facts: Protein: 0   Carbohydrates: 2.8 grams
Calories: 138

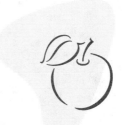

Peach Lemonade

    2 ounces light rum
    3 ounces sweet 'n' sour mix (sugar-free)
    ½ peach
    1 ounce peach sugar-free syrup

Combine all the ingredients in a blender with ice and blend until smooth. Pour into a wineglass.

Nutritional Facts: Protein: 0   Carbohydrates: 4.5 grams
Calories: 190

TROPICAL DRINKS

Frozen Mint Daiquiri

2½ ounces light rum
2 teaspoons Rose's Lime Juice
1 teaspoon Splenda® sweetener
6 mint leaves

Combine all the ingredients in a blender with ice and blend until smooth. Pour into a wineglass.

Nutritional Facts: Protein: 0   Carbohydrates: 1.4 grams
Calories: 199

Frozen Mint Julep

2 ounces bourbon
1 ounce lemon juice
1 ounce simple syrup (sugar-free)
6 mint leaves

Mix all the ingredients in a blender with ice and blend until smooth. Pour into a chilled cocktail glass.

Nutritional Facts: Protein: 0   Carbohydrates: 2.6 grams
Calories: 136

Piña Colada

    1 ounce light rum
    1 ounce dark rum
    2 ounces cream of coconut (sugar-free)
    1 ounce pineapple sugar-free syrup
    Pineapple wedge

Combine all the ingredients in a blender with ice and blend until smooth. Pour into a wineglass and serve with a straw. Garnish with the pineapple wedge.

Nutritional Facts: Protein: 0   Carbohydrates: 0   Calories: 230

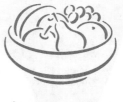

Strawberry Colada

    1 ounce light rum
    1 ounce dark rum
    2 ounces cream of coconut (sugar-free)
    1 ounce pineapple sugar-free syrup
    2 fresh or frozen strawberries
    Pineapple wedge

Combine all the ingredients in a blender with ice and blend until smooth. Pour into a wineglass and serve with a straw. Garnish with the pineapple wedge.

Nutritional Facts: Protein: 0   Carbohydrates: 2.5 grams
Calories: 160

Adult Hot Chocolate

 4 ounces half & half
 1 ounce vodka
 1 ounce chocolate sugar-free syrup
 $1/2$ ounce peppermint sugar-free syrup
 Whipped cream

Heat half & half and pour into an Irish coffee glass. Add vodka, chocolate sugar-free syrup and peppermint sugar-free syrup. Stir. Top with whipped cream.

Nutritional Facts: Protein: 4 grams   Carbohydrates: 5 grams
Calories: 345

Caribbean Coffee

 4 ounces half & half
 1 teaspoon Splenda® sweetener
 1 ounce dark rum
 1 ounce chocolate sugar-free syrup
 Whipped cream

Heat half & half and pour into an Irish coffee glass. Add Splenda® sweetener, rum and chocolate sugar-free syrup. Stir. Top with whipped cream.

Nutritional Facts: Protein: 4 grams   Carbohydrates: 5 grams
Calories: 345

DR. DOUGLAS J. MARKHAM

Coffee Lopez

6 ounces hot coffee
$^1/_2$ ounce cream of coconut (sugar-free)
$1^1/_2$ ounces Irish whisky
Whipped cream

Combine the hot coffee, cream of coconut and Irish whisky in an Irish coffee glass. Stir. Top with whipped cream.

Nutritional Facts: Protein: 2 grams   Carbohydrates: 2 grams
Calories: 146

Coffee Royale

1 teaspoon Splenda® sweetener
4 ounces hot coffee
2 ounces brandy
1 ounce heavy cream

Dissolve the Splenda® sweetener in hot coffee in an Irish coffee glass. Add brandy and heavy cream and stir. Top with whipped cream.

Nutritional Facts: Protein: 1 gram   Carbohydrates: 1 gram
Calories: 242

Endless Highway

  1 ounce bourbon
  1 ounce Irish cream sugar-free syrup
  2 ounces heavy cream
  4 ounces coffee

Mix ingredients into a coffee mug. Stir gently.

Nutritional Facts: Protein: 2 grams   Carbohydrates: 2 grams
Calories: 264

Hot Buttered Rum

  1 teaspoon Splenda® sweetener
  4 ounces boiling water
  2 ounces dark rum
  1 teaspoon butter
  1/4 teaspoon grated nutmeg

Dissolve the Splenda® sweetener into boiling water in an Irish coffee glass. Add the rum and butter and stir. Garnish with nutmeg on top.

Nutritional Facts: Protein: 0   Carbohydrates: 0   Calories: 130

Hot Coconut Coffee

  6 ounces hot coffee
  1 ounce rum
  1 ounce coconut sugar-free syrup
  Whipped cream

Combine the hot coffee, rum and coconut sugar-free syrup in an Irish coffee glass. Stir. Top with whipped cream.

Nutritional Facts: Protein: 0   Carbohydrates: 0   Calories: 65

Hot Toddy

  1 teaspoon Splenda® sweetener
  3 whole cloves
  1 cinnamon stick
  1 thin lemon slice
  4 ounces boiling water
  1 ounce bourbon
  Ground nutmeg

Put Splenda® sweetener, cloves, cinnamon stick and lemon slice into a coffee mug. Add 1 ounce boiling water, stir and let stand for 5 minutes. Add bourbon and 3 ounces boiling water and stir well. Sprinkle with ground nutmeg.

Nutritional Facts: Protein: 0   Carbohydrates: 0   Calories: 64

HOT DRINKS

Irish Coffee

1 teaspoon Splenda® sweetener
4 ounces hot coffee
1 ounce Irish whisky
1 ounce heavy cream

Dissolve the Splenda® sweetener into coffee in an Irish coffee glass. Add the whisky and stir. Add heavy cream on top.

Nutritional Facts: Protein: 1 gram   Carbohydrates: 1 gram
Calories: 164

Italian Coffee

$^{1}/_{2}$ ounce amaretto sugar-free syrup
4 ounces hot coffee
1 ounce brandy
1 ounce heavy cream

Combine sugar-free amaretto syrup and coffee in an Irish coffee glass. Add brandy and cream and stir.

Nutritional Facts: Protein: 1 gram   Carbohydrates: 1 gram
Calories: 171

Kentucky Coffee

6 ounces hot coffee
1¹/₂ ounces Kentucky bourbon
Whipped cream

Combine the hot coffee and Kentucky bourbon in an Irish coffee glass and stir. Top with whipped cream.

Nutritional Facts: Protein: 0   Carbohydrates: 0   Calories: 128

Kioki Coffee

6 ounces hot coffee
1 ounce brandy
1 ounce coffee or Kahlua® sugar-free syrup
Whipped cream

Combine the hot coffee, brandy and sugar-free Kahlua® syrup in an Irish coffee glass and stir. Top with whipped cream.

Nutritional Facts: Protein: 0   Carbohydrates: 0   Calories: 71

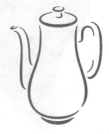

Mexican Coffee

  4 ounces hot coffee
  1 ounce vodka
  1 ounce coffee or Kahlua® sugar-free syrup
  2 ounces heavy cream

Combine the hot coffee, vodka and coffee or Kahlua® sugar-free syrup in an Irish coffee glass and stir. Add heavy cream on top.

Nutritional Facts: Protein: 2 grams   Carbohydrates: 2 grams
Calories: 265

Russian Coffee

  4 ounces hot coffee
  1 ounce vodka
  ½ ounce hazelnut sugar-free syrup
  ½ ounce heavy cream

Combine the hot coffee, vodka and hazelnut sugar-free syrup in an Irish coffee glass and stir. Add heavy cream on top.

Nutritional Facts: Protein: 1 gram   Carbohydrates: 1 gram
Calories: 115

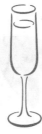

Venetian Coffee

6 ounces hot coffee
1 ounce brandy
1 teaspoon Splenda® sweetener
Whipped cream

Combine the hot coffee, brandy and Splenda® sweetener in an Irish coffee glass and stir. Top with whipped cream.

Nutritional Facts: Protein: 0   Carbohydrates: 0   Calories: 71

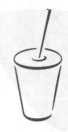

Nonalcoholic Drinks

Banana Smoothie

    1 ounce butter rum sugar-free syrup
    1 ounce banana sugar-free syrup
    1/2 ounce lime juice
    1/2 ounce yogurt
    1 teaspoon Splenda® sweetener

Combine all the ingredients in a blender with ice and blend until smooth. Pour into a wineglass.

Nutritional Facts: Protein: 1 gram   Carbohydrates: 3 grams Calories: 10

Big Banana

    4 ounces half & half
    1 ounce banana sugar-free syrup
    1/2 ounce coconut sugar-free syrup

Combine all the ingredients in a blender with ice and blend until smooth. Pour into a wineglass.

Nutritional Facts: Protein: 4 grams   Carbohydrates: 5 grams Calories: 280

Goddaughter

- 3 ounces cranberry juice (Ocean Spray® Light Cranberry Juice Cocktail)
- 3 ounces grapefruit juice (substitute Crystal Light® Ruby Red Grapefruit for grapefruit juice)

Shake all the ingredients in a shaker with ice and strain into a cocktail glass with ice.

Nutritional Facts: Protein: 0   Carbohydrates: 8.4 grams Calories: 15

Orange Fizz

- 3 ounces orange juice (substitute Sugar-Free Tang® for orange juice)
- 3 ounces diet ginger ale
- Orange slice
- 1 maraschino cherry

Pour the ingredients into a wineglass with ice and stir. Garnish with the orange slice and cherry.

Nutritional Facts: Protein: 0   Carbohydrates: 0   Calories: 0

Pippi Longstocking

    1 ounce green apple sugar-free syrup

    5 ounces diet ginger ale

    1 teaspoon grenadine (substitute cherry sugar-free syrup)

    1 teaspoon lemon juice

Pour the ingredients into a wineglass with ice and stir.

Nutritional Facts: Protein: 0   Carbohydrates: 0.6 grams
Calories: 2

Virgin Banana Colada

    1 ounce butter rum sugar-free syrup

    1 ounce pineapple sugar-free syrup

    2 ounces cream of coconut (sugar-free)

    1 ounce banana sugar-free syrup

    Cherry

Combine all the ingredients in a blender with ice and blend until smooth. Pour into a wineglass and garnish with the cherry.

Nutritional Facts: Protein: 2 grams   Carbohydrates: 2 grams
Calories: 50

Virgin Banana Daiquiri

- 1 ounce butter rum sugar-free syrup
- $^1/_2$ ounce triple sec (substitute orange sugar-free syrup)
- 1 ounce Rose's Lime Juice
- $^1/_2$ teaspoon Splenda® sweetener
- 1 ounce banana sugar-free syrup

Combine all the ingredients in a blender with ice and blend until smooth. Pour into a wineglass.

Nutritional Facts: Protein: 0   Carbohydrates: 2.8 grams
Calories: 8

Virgin Banana Foster

- 1 ounce butter rum sugar-free syrup
- 1 ounce banana sugar-free syrup
- 2 ounces heavy cream
- $^1/_2$ ounce vanilla sugar-free syrup

Combine all the ingredients in a blender with ice and blend until smooth. Pour into a wineglass.

Nutritional Facts: Protein: 2 grams   Carbohydrates: 2 grams
Calories: 200

Virgin Frozen Daiquiri

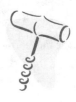

1 ounce butter rum sugar-free syrup
1 ounce Rose's Lime Juice
1 ounce orange sugar-free syrup
1 teaspoon Splenda® sweetener
Cherry

Combine all the ingredients in a blender with ice and blend until smooth. Pour into a wineglass and garnish with the cherry.

Nutritional Facts: Protein: 0   Carbohydrates: 2.8 grams
Calories: 8

Virgin Frozen Fruit Daiquiri

1 ounce butter rum sugar-free syrup
$^1/_2$ ounce sweet 'n' sour mix (sugar-free)
$^1/_2$ ounce heavy cream
1 ounce appropriate fruit-flavored sugar-free syrup (peach, strawberry, pineapple)
$^1/_4$ cup favorite fruit (peaches, strawberries, pineapple)

Combine all the ingredients in a blender with ice and blend until smooth. Pour into a wineglass.

Nutritional Facts: Protein: 1 gram   Carbohydrates: 5.5 grams
Calories: 110

Virgin Frozen Margarita

    4 ounces sweet 'n' sour mix (sugar-free)
    $^1/_2$ ounce orange sugar-free syrup
    Dash of Rose's Lime Juice
    Lime slice

Combine all the ingredients in a blender with ice and blend until smooth. Pour into a chilled cocktail glass and garnish with the lime slice.

Nutritional Facts: Protein: 0   Carbohydrates: 0   Calories: 0

Virgin Frozen Fruit Margarita

    3 ounces sweet 'n' sour mix (sugar-free)
    1 ounce appropriate fruit-flavored sugar-free syrup (peach, strawberry, pineapple)
    $^1/_4$ cup appropriate fruit (peaches, strawberries, pineapple)
    Dash of Rose's Lime Juice

Combine all the ingredients in a blender with ice and blend until smooth. Pour into a chilled cocktail glass.

Nutritional Facts: Protein: 0   Carbohydrates: 4.5 grams
Calories: 60

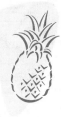

Virgin Frozen Matador

  2 ounces sweet 'n' sour mix (sugar-free)
  1 ounce pineapple sugar-free syrup
  2 teaspoons Rose's Lime Juice

Combine all the ingredients in a blender with ice and blend until smooth. Pour into a wineglass.

Nutritional Facts: Protein: 0   Carbohydrates: 1.4 grams
Calories: 4

Peach Lemonade

  1 ounce butter rum sugar-free syrup
  3 ounces sweet 'n' sour mix (sugar-free)
  ½ peach
  1 ounce peach sugar-free syrup

Combine all the ingredients in a blender with ice and blend until smooth. Pour into a wineglass.

Nutritional Facts: Protein: 0   Carbohydrates: 4.5 grams
Calories: 60

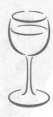

Shirley Temple

5½ ounces diet lemon-lime soda
1½ ounces grenadine (substitute cherry sugar-free syrup)
1 maraschino cherry

Pour the ingredients into a chilled cocktail glass with ice and stir. Garnish with the cherry.

Nutritional Facts: Protein: 0   Carbohydrates: 0   Calories: 0

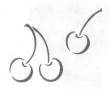

Virgin Frozen Mint Daiquiri

1 ounce butter rum sugar-free syrup
2 teaspoons Rose's Lime Juice
1 teaspoon Splenda® sweetener
6 mint leaves

Combine all the ingredients in a blender with ice and blend until smooth. Pour into a wineglass.

Nutritional Facts: Protein: 0   Carbohydrates: 1.4 grams
Calories: 4

Virgin Piña Colada

> 1 ounce butter rum sugar-free syrup
> 3 ounces cream of coconut (sugar-free)
> 1 ounce pineapple sugar-free syrup
> Pineapple wedge

Combine all the ingredients in a blender with ice and blend until smooth. Pour into a wineglass and serve with a straw. Garnish with the pineapple wedge.

Nutritional Facts: Protein: 2 grams   Carbohydrates: 2 grams
Calories: 100

Virgin Strawberry Colada

> 1 ounce butter rum sugar-free syrup
> 3 ounces cream of coconut (sugar-free)
> 1 ounce pineapple sugar-free syrup
> 2 fresh or frozen strawberries
> Pineapple wedge

Combine all the ingredients in a blender with ice and blend until smooth. Pour into a wineglass and serve with a straw. Garnish with the pineapple wedge.

Nutritional Facts: Protein: 2 grams   Carbohydrates: 4.5 grams
Calories: 120

Protein-Rich Low-Carb Snacks

Snacks Requiring No Recipes

- Cream cheese (no fat or low fat) and caviar on cucumber slices
- Smoked salmon on cucumber slices
- Baked Brie cheese wheel
- Premium domestic and/or imported cheese
- Peanuts
- Cashews
- Mixed nuts
- Smoked almonds
- Roasted hazelnuts
- Macadamia nuts
- Pumpkin seeds
- Sunflower seeds
- Tapenades (mushrooms, olives, and artichokes)
- Jumbo shrimp
- Pepperoni slices
- Spicy sausages
- Chilled oysters on the half shell
- Smoked oysters

- Chicken, turkey or ham slices, rolled up with softened cream cheese in the center
- Assorted cheese and fruit platter
- Antipasto platter (sliced cheeses, salami, marinated mushrooms, artichoke hearts and olives, arranged artistically on a platter)

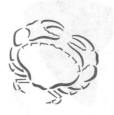

Dips and Dippers

Dip suggestions: Choose one of the following recipes, your favorite low-carb dressings or prepared dips such as blue cheese dressing, ranch dressing, French onion dip, spinach dip, etc.

Dipper suggestions: artichokes, asparagus spears, broccoli, cauliflower, zucchini, celery, sliced cucumbers, bell peppers, mushrooms and radishes.

Note: Nutritional facts will not be listed for dips. Be aware that certain dips do include protein, carbohydrates and calories. Dips are intended to coat your dippers to enhance their taste and not meant for a meal replacement.

Artichoke Dip

   1 (14-ounce) can artichoke hearts, drained, and blended
      or chopped
   1 cup mayonnaise (no fat or low fat)
   1 cup Parmesan cheese
   1/2 teaspoon garlic powder or 1 clove garlic, minced

Preheat oven to 350°F. Mix all ingredients. Pour into 9-inch pie pan and bake 20 minutes or until lightly browned.

Crabmeat Dip

   1/2 cup butter
   8 ounces cream cheese (no fat or low fat)
   1 (6 1/2-ounce) can crabmeat
   1 tablespoon grated onion
   2 to 3 dashes of Worcestershire sauce
   Salt, to taste

Melt butter and cheese in top of double boiler. Add crabmeat and its juice. Stir thoroughly. Add remaining ingredients and serve hot.

Onion Dip

   1 1/2 cups sour cream (no fat or low fat)
   2 tablespoons dry onion soup mix
   2 ounces crumbled blue cheese
   1/3 cup chopped walnuts

Thoroughly combine the sour cream with the onion mix. Stir in remaining ingredients.

Cheese Fondue Dip

2 (10³/₄-ounce) cans condensed cheese soup
2 cups grated sharp cheddar cheese
1 tablespoon Worcestershire sauce
1 teaspoon lemon juice
1 package freeze-dried or fresh chives

Combine condensed soup, grated cheese, Worcestershire sauce, lemon juice and chives. Cover and heat on low in Crock-Pot for 2 to 2¹/₂ hours. Stir until smooth and well blended. Keep hot in the Crock-Pot.

Spinach Dip

1 package frozen chopped spinach
1 cup mayonnaise (no fat or low fat)
1 (8-ounce) can water chestnuts, chopped
3 green onions, finely chopped
1 cup sour cream (no fat or low fat)
1 packet dry vegetable soup mix

Defrost, drain and squeeze moisture from the spinach. Combine with remaining ingredients. Chill several hours.

Cocktail Sauce

  1 cup catsup
  1–2 tablespoons horseradish (to taste)
  1 tablespoon lemon juice
  $1/2$ teaspoon Worcestershire sauce
  $1/4$ teaspoon salt
  Dash of pepper

Mix all ingredients and chill.

Clam Dip

  8 ounces cream cheese, softened
  $1/2$ cup sour cream
  1 (6-ounce) can clams, minced (reserve 2 tablespoons of juice)
  1 tablespoon fresh parsley, chopped
  1 clove garlic, minced
  $1/4$ teaspoon Worcestershire sauce

In a small bowl, beat cheese, sour cream, and reserved 2 table-spoons of clam juice until smooth and well blended. Stir in remaining ingredients. Cover and refrigerate.

DIPS AND DIPPERS

Avocado and Crabmeat

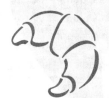

- 1 avocado
- 1 (6-ounce) can crabmeat
- 3 scallions, finely chopped
- 1 tablespoon mayonnaise
- 1 teaspoon olive oil
- ½ teaspoon nutmeg
- ½ teaspoon salt
- ½ teaspoon pepper
- ½ teaspoon paprika

Chop avocado and add the crabmeat, scallions, mayonnaise, oil and nutmeg. Sprinkle with salt and pepper. Mix and serve in a cocktail glass over ice, sprinkled with paprika.

Nutritional Facts: Protein: 14 grams   Carbohydrates: 5 grams

Bacon Wrapped Water Chestnuts

- 1 pound bacon
- 2 cans whole water chestnuts

Heat oven to 325°F. Wrap half piece of bacon around each water chestnut and spear with a toothpick. Place on a foil-lined cookie sheet and bake 1 hour. Transfer to paper towel–lined platter. Serve warm.

Nutritional Facts: Protein: 3.5 grams   Carbohydrates: 1 gram

Baked Buffalo Wings

2 tablespoons melted butter

1/4 cup hot pepper sauce

2 tablespoons rice vinegar

30 chicken drumettes or 18 small drumsticks

Paprika for sprinkling

Preheat oven to 350°F. Lightly oil a baking sheet. Mix together butter, hot pepper sauce and vinegar. Dip chicken into mixture, then place on baking sheet. Sprinkle lightly with paprika. Bake until crisp and brown (about 30 minutes).

Nutritional Facts: Protein: 7 grams   Carbohydrates: 1 gram

Beef Roll-Ups

1 ounce thinly sliced roast beef

Stuffed green olives

Wrap each slice of beef around a stuffed green olive and serve.

Nutritional Facts: Protein: 7 grams   Carbohydrates: 1 gram

Crab Stuffed Mushrooms

    8 ounces cream cheese, softened to room temperature
    1 tablespoon chopped green onion
    ½ cup crabmeat, drained and flaked
    ½ teaspoon Worcestershire sauce
    ½ pound fresh mushrooms, cleaned, with stems removed
    ¼ cup grated Parmesan cheese

Preheat oven to 350°F. In a mixing bowl, combine all ingredients except for mushrooms and Parmesan cheese. Stuff mushrooms with crab mixture, mounding the tops slightly. Sprinkle with Parmesan cheese. Bake until filling is golden (about 20 minutes).

Nutritional Facts: Protein: 2 grams   Carbohydrates: 1 gram

Ceviche

2½ cups lemon juice

1½ cups Rose's Lime Juice

1 tablespoon white pepper

1 tablespoon salt

1 tablespoon granulated garlic

1 ounce Tabasco

2 ounces safflower oil

5 pounds Pacific red snapper (cut into ½-inch cubes)

½ bunch diced green onions or scallions

½ bunch fresh cilantro (chopped)

1 medium bell pepper (diced)

In a large bowl, combine lemon and lime juices. Then add white pepper, salt, garlic, Tabasco and safflower oil. Mix well. Add the cubed red snapper, onions, cilantro and bell pepper. Gently mix well. Refrigerate for 12 hours to blend flavors before serving. Serve on chilled bed of lettuce, with slices of lemon and a side dish of your favorite salsa.

Nutritional Facts: Protein: 10 grams   Carbohydrates: 2 grams

Deviled Eggs

6 hard-cooked eggs
$1/4$ teaspoon salt
$1/2$ teaspoon dry mustard
$1/4$ teaspoon pepper
$1/4$ cup mayonnaise
Paprika

Cut peeled eggs lengthwise and scoop out yolks. Mix yolks with above ingredients and blend well. Fill whites with mixture, cover and refrigerate until ready to serve. Sprinkle with paprika.

Nutritional Facts: Protein: 3.5 grams   Carbohydrates: 0

Ham Roll-Ups

1 ounce thinly sliced ham
1 ounce squares cheddar or Swiss cheese

Slice thin strips of ham and wrap around cheese squares. Use favorite mustard for dipping.

Nutritional Facts: Protein: 14 grams   Carbohydrates: 0

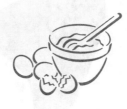

Herb Olives

2 cups unpitted ripe or green olives

2 small hot, dried red chilies

2 cloves garlic

2 tablespoons finely chopped celery leaves

2 tablespoons drained capers

12 rosemary leaves

1 bay leaf

1 cup olive oil

Place olives in a jar, interspersed with all the ingredients except oil. Pour in enough oil to cover olives. Cover jar and shake well. Refrigerate 3 or 4 days before using; shake jar several times during this time. Remove garlic if olives are stored for any length of time.

Nutritional Facts: Protein: 0   Carbohydrates: 1 gram

Jiffy Tomato Stack Ups

3 large tomatoes

Salt

4 ounces Swiss cheese, shredded

10-ounce package chopped broccoli, cooked and drained

$^1/_4$ cup chopped onion

Cut tomatoes into slices about $^3/_4$-inch thick. Sprinkle each lightly with salt. Set aside 2 tablespoons of the shredded cheese; combine remaining cheese, broccoli and onion. Place tomato slices on greased baking sheet. Spoon broccoli mixture onto tomatoes. Sprinkle with reserved cheese. Broil 7 to 8 inches from heat for 10 to 12 minutes or till cheese bubbles and tomato slices are hot.

Nutritional Facts: Protein: 6.5 grams   Carbohydrates: 6.6 grams

Salmon-Stuffed Avocados

8 ounces cream cheese, softened
2 (7½-ounce) cans salmon, drained
2 teaspoons Worcestershire sauce
1½ teaspoons salt
⅛ teaspoon pepper
3 avocados, black- or green-skinned
1 tablespoon lemon juice

In large bowl, with wooden spoon, beat the cream cheese with the salmon, Worcestershire, salt and pepper until fluffy. Halve avocados lengthwise; remove pits. Brush cut sides with lemon juice to prevent discoloration. Fill hollow of each half with cream cheese mixture. Refrigerate until well chilled, about 1 hour.

Nutritional Facts: Protein: 11 grams   Carbohydrates: 5 grams

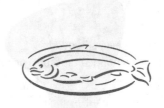

Smoked Salmon Rolls

4 ounces cream cheese
1 tablespoon lemon juice
1 tablespoon grated onion
Freshly ground black pepper
2 slices smoked salmon or 1 can smoked salmon
Chopped parsley

Have cheese at room temperature and mix in lemon juice, grated onion and a little pepper. Blend until very soft. Spread on slices of salmon, roll up like a Swiss roll and cut into 2-inch pieces. Chill several hours before serving. Dip both ends of the rolls in chopped parsley.

Nutritional Facts: Protein: 6 grams   Carbohydrates: 1 gram

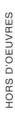

Swedish Meatballs

½ cup fresh bread crumbs
1 pound ground round
½ pound ground pork shoulder
1 egg
1 cup milk (no fat or low fat)
1 onion, minced
1 teaspoon Splenda® sweetener
½ teaspoon allspice
½ teaspoon nutmeg
Salt
Pepper
Safflower oil

Sauce:

1 cup sour cream
¼ cup flour
¼ teaspoon nutmeg

Mix together all ingredients except oil. Brown 1-inch balls in oil. Drain and discard excess fat from the skillet. Set meatballs in a serving dish.

To make the sauce, add the sour cream, flour and nutmeg to a skillet and beat with a whisk until dissolved and warmed.

Serve sauce with meatballs or pour sauce over meatballs and serve in a chafing dish.

Nutritional Facts: Protein: 7 grams   Carbohydrates: 2 grams

Sweet and Sour Meatballs

2 pounds lean ground beef
2 eggs, slightly beaten
1/2 cup bread crumbs
1/2 cup water
Salt, to taste
Pepper, to taste
Garlic powder, to taste
1 (12-ounce) bottle chili sauce
1/2 cup grape sugar-free jelly
Juice of 1 lemon

Combine ground beef, eggs, bread crumbs, water, salt, pepper and garlic powder. Shape into walnut-size balls. Combine chili sauce, grape jelly and lemon in large saucepan. Heat until jelly melts. Drop uncooked meatballs into sauce and simmer for 45 minutes. Serve in a chafing dish.

Nutritional Facts: Protein: 7 grams   Carbohydrates: 3 grams

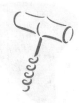

Sweet and Sour Smoky Sausages

8 ounces little smoky sausages
$^1/_2$ cup vinegar
$^1/_2$ cup Splenda® sweetener
$^1/_4$ cup sherry wine
1 tablespoon soy sauce
1 teaspoon grated fresh ginger root
2 teaspoons cornstarch
1 tablespoon water
1 (10-ounce) can pineapple chunks, drained
1 green pepper, cut into 1-inch squares
$^1/_2$ cup maraschino cherries, drained

Brown sausages. Drain on paper towels. Boil together briefly vinegar, Splenda® sweetener, sherry, soy sauce and ginger. Blend cornstarch and water together and add to above mixture. Cook until transparent. Add sausages, pineapple, green pepper and cherries and slowly heat. Serve in a chafing dish.

Nutritional Facts: Protein: 3.5 grams   Carbohydrates: 2 grams

Turkey Roll-Ups

    1 ounce of turkey
    1 green olive
    Pinch of pimentos

A great way to use leftover holiday turkey. Slice turkey into thin strips. Wrap around small green olives stuffed with pimentos and spear with toothpicks. Ready for dipping into your favorite sauce.

Nutritional Facts: Protein: 7 grams   Carbohydrates: 1 gram

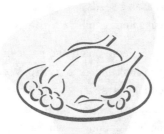

Zucchini-Cheese Squares

1 small onion, chopped
1 clove garlic, minced
2$\frac{1}{2}$ cups shredded zucchini
6 eggs, beaten
$\frac{1}{3}$ cup bread crumbs
$\frac{1}{2}$ teaspoon salt
$\frac{1}{2}$ teaspoon basil
$\frac{1}{2}$ teaspoon oregano
$\frac{1}{4}$ teaspoon pepper
3 cups shredded cheddar cheese
$\frac{1}{2}$ cup grated Parmesan cheese
$\frac{1}{4}$ cup toasted sesame seeds
$\frac{1}{2}$ cup olive oil or safflower oil

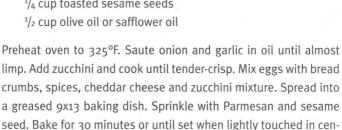

Preheat oven to 325°F. Saute onion and garlic in oil until almost limp. Add zucchini and cook until tender-crisp. Mix eggs with bread crumbs, spices, cheddar cheese and zucchini mixture. Spread into a greased 9x13 baking dish. Sprinkle with Parmesan and sesame seed. Bake for 30 minutes or until set when lightly touched in center. Cool at least 15 minutes. Cut into 1-inch squares and serve warm, room temperature or cold.

Nutritional Facts: Protein: 2 grams   Carbohydrates: 1 gram

Index

INDEX

INDEX